Single-Session Therapy and Its Future

Single-Session Therapy and Its Future provides an introduction to the major principles of single-session therapy and what currently constitutes good practice in the field.

The book is a timely reflection on where SST is at, and where it might be heading. It is comprised of interviews with well-known leaders and experts in this field, outlining what they think will happen, hope will happen and fear might happen as the future of SST unfolds. The book further notes the growth and development of SST in many different contexts internationally in the past 30 years.

The book will be of interest to practitioners with little knowledge/ experience of the SST "mindset" or mode of service delivery, as well as seasoned SST practitioners. It will also appeal to practitioners working with many client groups around the world.

Windy Dryden, PhD, is Emeritus Professor of Psychotherapeutic Studies at Goldsmiths, University of London and is an international authority on Rational Emotive Behaviour Therapy (REBT) and Single-Session Therapy (SST). He has worked in psychotherapy for over 45 years and is the author and editor of over 235 books.

Routledge Focus on Mental Health

Routledge Focus on Mental Health presents short books on current topics, linking in with cutting-edge research and practice.

For a full list of titles in this series, please visit www.routledge.com/Routledge-Focus-on-Mental-Health/book-series/RFMH

Single-Session Therapy and Its Future

What SST Leaders Think

Windy Dryden

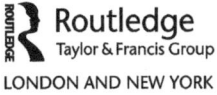

Routledge
Taylor & Francis Group

LONDON AND NEW YORK

First published 2021
by Routledge
2 Park Square, Milton Park, Abingdon, Oxon OX14 4RN

and by Routledge
52 Vanderbilt Avenue, New York, NY 10017

Routledge is an imprint of the Taylor & Francis Group, an informa business

© 2021 Windy Dryden

British Library Cataloguing-in-Publication Data
A catalogue record for this book is available from the British Library

Library of Congress Cataloging-in-Publication Data
Names: Dryden, Windy, author.
Title: Single-session therapy and its future : what sst
leaders think / Windy Dryden, Ph.D.
Description: Milton Park, Abingdon, Oxon ; New York, NY : Routledge, 2021. |
Series: Routledge focus on mental health |
Includes bibliographical references and index. |
Identifiers: LCCN 2020037320 (print) |
LCCN 2020037321 (ebook) | ISBN 9780367616519 (hardback) |
ISBN 9780367616526 (paperback) | ISBN 9781003105862 (ebook)
Subjects: LCSH: Single-session psychotherapy. | Psychotherapist and patient.
Classification: LCC RC480.55 .D768 2021 (print) |
LCC RC480.55 (ebook) | DDC 616.89/14–dc23
LC record available at https://lccn.loc.gov/2020037320
LC ebook record available at https://lccn.loc.gov/2020037321

ISBN: 978-0-367-61651-9 (hbk)
ISBN: 978-1-003-10586-2 (ebk)

Typeset in Sabon
by Newgen Publishing UK

Contents

Acknowledgements

I wish to thank Michael Hoyt, Moshe Talmon and Jeffrey Young for allowing me to interview them and for letting me use these interviews in this book.

I wish to thank the British Psychological Society, Guilford Press and Taylor & Francis for granting me permission to publish Chapters 2, 3 and 4 respectively.

- Chapter 2 originally appeared as Dryden, W. (2019). It forced me to think in different ways about single session therapy. *The Psychologist, 32*(11), 44–46.
- Chapter 3 originally appeared as Hoyt, M.F., & Dryden, W. (2018). Toward the future of single-session therapy: An interview. *Journal of Systemic Therapies, 37*(1), 79–89.
- Chapter 4 originally appeared as Young, J., & Dryden, W. (2019). Single-session therapy – past and future: An interview. *British Journal of Guidance and Counselling, 47*(5), 645–654.

Preface

In 1990, Moshe Talmon wrote an important book on single-session therapy which provided a foundation for subsequent developments in SST and its applications to many client groups in many contexts around the world (see Chapter 2). Three International Symposia on Single-Session Therapy and Walk-In Services – in Melbourne, Australia, in 2012 (Hoyt & Talmon, 2014), in Banff in Canada in 2015 (Hoyt, Bobele, Slive, Young & Talmon, 2018), and again in Melbourne, Australia, in 2019 – provide testimony to the creativity of those who have drawn on Talmon's pioneering work and challenged traditional ideas about the nature, practice and length of therapy.

My own interest in SST came from the many demos of therapy that I have done over the years. Whenever I give a training course, I do a demonstration session of therapy and I came to realise that these sessions were examples of SST and ones that took place in 30 minutes or less. Looking for a new challenge when I retired from my university post, I re-read Talmon's (1990) book and got enthused by the possibilities. Based on his and others' writings, I developed a single-session-based approach to CBT which I called 'Single-Session Integrated CBT' (Dryden, 2017) and which can be used in the NHS as well as in private practice. Indeed, my view is that if the NHS really wanted to improve access to psychological treatment, then it would offer a nationwide set of walk-in clinics staffed by people keen to help individuals as quickly as possible at the point of need (an hour after attending a walk-in clinic) rather than, at present, at the point of availability (often months after a person has consulted their GP).

In 2018, while writing my general book on SST (Dryden, 2019), I decided to interview three of the leaders of the single-session therapy community (Moshe Talmon, Michael Hoyt and Jeffrey Young) about the future of this exciting field. Such was the richness of the material I gathered during these interviews that I decided to bring them together in one place so that those interested in SST can read and study what these leaders think will happen, hope will happen and fear might happen as the future of SST unfolds.

To put these interviews in context I have written an introduction to SST discussing the ideas that underpin SST and what constitutes good practice. This chapter seeks to define the present of SST. Our experts offer their ideas about its future.

References

Dryden, W. (2017). *Single-Session Integrated CBT (SSI-CBT)*. Abingdon, Oxon: Routledge.

Dryden, W. (2019). *Single-Session Therapy: 100 Key Points and Techniques*. Abingdon, Oxon: Routledge.

Hoyt, M.F., Bobele, M., Slive, A., Young, J., & Talmon, M. (Eds.) (2018). *Single-Session Therapy by Walk-In or Appointment: Administrative, Clinical, and Supervisory Aspects of One-At-A-Time Services*. New York: Routledge.

Hoyt, M.F., & Talmon, M.F. (Eds.) (2014). *Capturing the Moment: Single Session Therapy and Walk-In Services*. Bethel, CT: Crown House Publishing.

Talmon, M. (1990). *Single Session Therapy: Maximizing the Effect of the First (and Often Only) Therapeutic Encounter*. San Francisco, CA: Jossey-Bass.

Windy Dryden, London & Eastbourne
March 2020

Chapter 1

Single-session therapy (SST)

An introduction

Overview

In this chapter, I provide an introduction to the major principles of single-session therapy and what constitutes good practice in this field.[1] In particular, I show how SST can be used to help meet client need where the demand for services outstrips supply.

I begin by providing some relevant definitions before considering the foundations of SST. I then compare the features of help provided at the point of need and the features of help provided at the point of availability. It is clear from this comparison that SST is consistent with the former. I go on to consider the question of whether SST is a mindset, a mode of service delivery or a discrete therapeutic approach, arguing that it is the first two and not the latter. I then discuss the goals of SST, before considering the issue of indications and contraindications for SST. There follows a comprehensive discussion of the Dos and Don'ts of good practice in SST, before I provide an example of an effective single-session structure. I end the chapter by considering and responding to common misconceptions of SST.

Introduction

Imagine this scenario. Samantha Smith has been struggling with problems of anxiety for several months and, after prompting from her family, she decides to see her GP. When she telephones for an appointment, she is given one seven days hence. At the consultation, her GP agrees that Samantha could benefit from 'talking therapy' and gives her details of the local IAPT[2] service and asks her to make contact. She telephones the IAPT service the same day, and a receptionist arranges for a psychological wellbeing practitioner (PWP) to carry out a telephone assessment with Samantha which will take place in ten days.

This assessment takes place, and the PWP concludes that Samantha is suffering from mild to moderate generalised anxiety disorder (GAD) and refers her for low-intensity CBT which will either take the form of guided self-help or occur in a psychoeducational group. There will be a four-week wait for such help. If Samantha's GAD was assessed to be in the severe range, then she would have been referred for high-intensity CBT which would occur in a one-to-one setting and for which there would be an eight-week wait. Samantha was reluctant to opt for guided self-help and did not want to join a group. She preferred to see a therapist one-to-one. The PWP told Samantha that he would have to make a special case for this to his supervisor and that he would contact her in one week. He did so and told Samantha that her request for one-to-one therapy was granted and she was offered an appointment in eight weeks. The time it took for Samantha to have her first therapy session after seeing her GP was eleven and a half weeks.

Contrast this with what would happen if Samantha went to an agency that offers a walk-in option. She would decide that she wanted to talk to a mental health professional, she would 'walk in' to the service, complete a brief one-to-two page intake form and then have a session, usually less than an hour after arrival.

This chapter is based on the second approach to service delivery rather than the first.

Some definitions

Let me begin by defining some important terms.

Single-session therapy

There are three main approaches to defining single-session therapy. I will deal with them one at a time.

The 'Ronseal' definition

It may be thought that it is clear what single-session therapy (SST) is. It is therapy that lasts for a single session. This is what I call the

'Ronseal' definition of SST.[3] Using the 'Ronseal' definition we can distinguish between two types of SST. First, there is therapy that is designed to last for a single session which is known in the SST literature as single-session therapy 'by design'. Then there is therapy that lasts for a single session because the client unilaterally decides to attend for only one session. This is known as single-session therapy 'by default' in the SST literature.

Moshe Talmon's definition

Single-session therapy is not a new concept in the psychotherapy literature. Indeed, Sigmund Freud published details of two single-session therapies that he carried out, one with Aurelia Öhm-Kronich – better known as 'Katharina' (Freud & Breuer, 1895) and the other with Gustav Mahler (Kuehn, 1965). However, the recent interest in SST can be traced to the publication of a book by the Israeli clinical psychologist Moshe Talmon (1990), based on research he conducted whilst working in northern California, entitled *Single Session Therapy: Maximizing the Effect of the First (and Often Only) Therapeutic Encounter*.

In his book, Talmon (1990: xv) defined single-session therapy 'as one face-to-face meeting between a therapist and a patient with no previous or subsequent sessions within one year' (Talmon, 1990: xv). According to this definition, telephone intake and follow-up are deemed to be part of SST as they do not take place face-to-face. Twenty-eight years later, Hoyt, Bobele, Slive, Young and Talmon (2018a: 18) reported that this 'SST definition of *no other sessions in the year before or after* is, of course, arbitrary and was used for research purposes'.

One session, possibly more

Perhaps the most accepted view of single-session therapy has been concisely put forward by Weir, Wills, Young and Perlesz (2008: 12), who said SST 'is not a "one-off" therapy but rather a structured first session which attempts to maximise the client's first therapeutic encounter, understanding that it may be the only appointment the client chooses to attend, while entertaining the possibility of ongoing work'. The elements that are important here are that i) both therapist and client will try to get the work done in the first session and

ii) there is agreement that more therapy is available if the client needs it. This definition emphasises the deliberate nature of SST. It is something that is agreed in advance by the therapist and the client. As Hymmen, Stalker and Cait (2013: 61) have written: 'SST refers to a conscious approach to make the most of the first session knowing it may be the only session the client decides to attend—not to the situation where there is an expectation that the client will attend multiple sessions but chooses to attend just one.' Regardless of definition, it is clear that the practice of SST is growing internationally and that it is being applied to a wider range of problems (Hoyt & Dryden, 2018).

One-at-a-time therapy (OAATT)

One-at-a-time therapy (OAATT) is a term that was coined by Michael Hoyt (2011) and elaborated by Slive and Bobele (2011, 2014) to describe the situation where therapy takes place one contact at a time, and one contact may be all the time that is needed. While additional sessions may be available if needed, OAATT precludes the possibility of clients booking a block of sessions in advance. I have stressed that to help the client get the most out of the first session in OAATT the therapist needs to encourage them to go away and reflect on what they got from the session, digest it as fully as possible, act on what was learned and let time pass before deciding whether or not to book a further session of therapy. In my view, this 'reflection–digestion–action–let time pass' process is key to OAATT (Dryden, 2019a).

The foundations of SST

Every approach to therapy and service provision is founded on a set of assumptions and/or principles. In this section, I will outline a number of such foundations of single-session therapy.

Jeff Young's 'three findings' foundations

Jeff Young (2018), a major developer of SST in Australia, notes that the term 'single-session therapy' (SST) is an inaccurate one, but one that should be retained because of its ability to shock and stimulate discussion. Thus, SST challenges generally held beliefs about therapy such as i) 'more is better', ii) real change happens slowly and gradually and iii) effective therapy is built upon the therapeutic relationship, which takes time to develop.

However, rather than define SST, Young (2018) outlines three findings that serve as some of its foundations. These findings are:

> Finding #1: the most common number of service contacts that clients attend is one, followed by two, followed by three… irrespective of diagnosis, complexity, or the severity of their problem (Talmon, 1990).
>
> Finding #2: the majority (often about 70–80%) of those people who attend only one session, across a range of therapies, report that the single session was adequate given their current circumstance (Talmon, 1990; Bloom, 2001; Campbell, 2012).
>
> Finding #3: it seems impossible to accurately predict who will attend only one session and who will attend more, a proposition that has significant clinical and organizational ramifications. If it cannot be predicted who will attend only one session and who will attend more, it follows that both possibilities need to be embraced simultaneously by both the worker and by their service system. That is, the first session should logically be conducted 'as if' it may also be the last.
>
> (Young, 2018: 44)

Other foundations

In addition to the above three findings, the following also serve as foundations of SST.

Even a brief encounter can be therapeutic

In life, we meet numerous people and most of these we will not see again. Occasionally, such 'brief encounters' can have a therapeutic impact on us, which may even last a lifetime. My own therapeutic 'brief encounter' came from listening to a radio interview with Michael Bentine, the British comedian, when I was in my mid-teens. Like me, Bentine had a stammer and, during that interview, he was asked how he coped with stammering. He replied that he learned to develop the attitude 'If I stammer, I stammer. Too bad!' which helped him with his anxiety about speaking in public. I really resonated with this attitude, and I have been applying it for almost 50 years. So, a 30-second segment from a radio interview half a century ago had an ongoing positive effect on me. The fact that it is possible that a brief therapy encounter can have a positive impact on a client is an important foundation of SST

Therapy length is expandable

Parkinson's law of psychotherapy states that therapy expands and contracts to fill the time allocated to it (Appelbaum, 1975). Taking this law, Talmon (1993: 135) observed that: 'When the therapist and client expect change to happen now, it often does.' This principle is an important foundation of SST.

Human beings have the capability to help themselves quickly under specific circumstances

If human beings could only change slowly, then single-session therapy and one-at-a-time therapy would not have been developed, let alone would they have flourished. For change to occur quickly, three conditions need to be met: i) knowledge of what to do to bring about change, ii) having a committed reason to change and iii) being prepared to accept the costs of change.

Albert Ellis in his clinical seminars once referred to the case of 'Vera'. 'Vera' sought help for elevator phobia and joined one of Ellis's groups because she could not afford individual therapy. Over the next few years, despite knowing what she needed to do to address her problem (condition i), she did not do so because she lacked a good enough reason to change (condition ii). Then, one Friday afternoon, 'Vera' booked an individual session with Ellis which was unheard of. She told Ellis that the office where she worked was being moved on Monday morning from the fifth floor, which she could walk up to, to the 105th floor, which she obviously couldn't! As she needed her job, she now had a committed reason to change quickly. She had to be over her phobia by Monday morning! Ellis responded that she knew what she had to do – ride elevators repeatedly over the weekend and tolerate the great discomfort of doing so (condition iii). This is exactly what 'Vera' did and she was over her phobia by Sunday night. She changed because she met all three conditions outlined above.

Much can be achieved if certain conditions are present

These conditions are:

The client is ready to change, and the therapist can capitalise on their readiness. As can be seen from the above, much can be achieved if the client is ready to change. However, it is also important that the therapist can respond to that state of readiness and help the client to capitalise on it. The old adage 'it takes two to tango' is particularly apt here.

The therapist and client share realistic expectations for client change. The therapeutic dyad should expect neither quantum change (i.e. sudden, dramatic and enduring transformations that affect a broad range of personal emotion, cognition and behaviour) nor no change. Realistic expectations for change in SST include becoming unstuck and taking a few steps towards goal achievement and making a plan to sustain this change (see the section on the goals of SST below).

The therapist and client embark intentionally on SST. Initially, Talmon (1990) reported on the situation where he followed up 200 cases from his work at the Kaiser Permanente clinic in northern California. These were clients who only attended for a single session although Talmon thought they would attend for more. As we have seen, this is known as SST by default. Most client benefit, however, is likely to occur when the therapist and the client embark on SST intentionally. As mentioned before, this is known as SST by design.

SST reflects what a lot of clients or service users want from therapy agencies

In addition to the finding that the modal number of sessions that clients have internationally is '1', feedback from service users indicates that what they want is in keeping with what SST has to offer.

Here is an example from a group of service users from an NHS trust in north-east England. This group said that they wanted

- clarity on what is on offer
- therapists to be realistic and not overstate choice
- therapists not to offer very long-term therapy which feels overwhelming but to offer short-term pieces of work which

are reviewed so that the person can 'get out' without causing offence if that is what they want

- less therapy, but timely
- therapists to link all the bits of the system together rather than therapy being removed from other work.

The therapist structures the session effectively

The SST therapist tends to bring to the work certain ideas about the session that help both them and their client get the most from the session. Thus, the effective SST therapist tends to view the session as complete in itself and plans the session according to the time available. However, most importantly, they have in mind a structure to the session that is flexible enough to incorporate modifications as needed. Hoyt (2000, 2018) has outlined one such structure. He argues that a single session has five phases: i) *a pre-session phase* where induction and seeding occur; ii) *an early phase* where alliance-building occurs, any pre-treatment change is discussed and built upon, and goal-setting takes place; iii) *a middle phase* where a change-based refocusing is facilitated, and solutions for change are discussed, selected and rehearsed; iv) *a late phase* where action planning is done, relapse prevention occurs, and leave-taking takes place – this termination phase is where the possibility of future sessions is discussed – and v) *a follow-through phase* where follow-up and evaluation take place and the client returns for more help if needed.

Help provided at the point of need vs at the point of availability

One of the objectives of this chapter is to make a case for providing help at the point of client need. At the outset, I outlined two types of help provision: help at the point of need and help at the point of availability. Table 1.1 details more clearly the differences between the two. It is quite apparent from this table that SST practitioners are best placed to provide help at the point of client need.

SST: mindset and mode of service delivery rather than a therapeutic approach

Most people in the SST field hold the view that SST is a mindset and/or a mode of service delivery and is definitely not a specific

Table 1.1 **Differences between help at the point of need and help at the point of availability**

Help at the point of need	Help at the point of availability
• It is better to respond to client need by providing some help straightaway rather than by waiting to provide the best possible help.	• It is better to have clients wait for the best possible help than to provide them with some help when they need it.
• Providing immediate help is more important than carrying out an assessment.	• Carrying out an assessment is more important than offering immediate help.
• Therapy should start immediately. A case formulation should be carried out only if needed.	• Therapy should only be carried out on the basis of a formulation of the case.
• Therapy can be initiated in the absence of a case history.	• It is important to take a case history before therapy is initiated.
• People have the resources to make use of help provided at the point of need.	• People have the resources to make use of help provided on the basis of a case formulation.
• Sooner is better.	• More is better.
• The best way to see if a client will respond well to therapy is by offering them therapy and seeing how they respond.	• The best way to see if a client will respond well to therapy is to offer them the most appropriate therapy based on a full assessment of their problems and on a formulation of their 'case'.
• Therapy can be initiated and risk managed if this becomes an issue.	• Risk has to be properly managed before therapy is initiated.
• Appropriate therapy length is best determined by the client.	• Appropriate therapy length is best determined by the therapist.
• When a person does not return for another session, this may well indicate that the person is satisfied with what they achieved, although it may be the case that they were dissatisfied with the help provided.	• When a person does not return for another session or before they have completed their 'course of treatment', they have dropped out of this treatment and it should be regarded as a bad outcome.

therapeutic approach. Thus, SST can be practised by therapists from a broad spectrum of therapeutic approaches (Hoyt & Talmon, 2014a; Hoyt et al., 2018b; Dryden, 2019b).

The SST mindset

Jeff Young (2018) has outlined the features of this mindset or what he terms 'an SST-informed attitude to clinical work'. These features are:

- approaching the first session 'as if' it could be the last, irrespective of diagnosis, complexity or severity
- exploring what each client wants to walk away with at the end of the session at hand (rather than the usual question of what the client wants from a course of therapy)
- prioritising what to focus on – negotiated between client and clinician, but largely client led
- checking in at various points throughout the session to ensure the work is on track
- sharing directly, albeit in a tentative way, feedback, advice, strategies, commendations and information that the clinician feels is helpful, driven by the idea 'what would I want to share with this client if I never see them again?'
- providing resources and clarifying next steps.

The paradoxical nature of the SST mindset

Therapists need to understand that a key aspect of the SST mindset is its paradoxical nature. Thus, when clients know that more sessions are available, they are more likely to be satisfied with one session knowing that they *could* return later if necessary. Michael Hoyt, one of the field's leading figures, has written eloquently on what happens when a one-session-only approach to SST is taken:

> Insistence produces resistance, imposition produces opposition, push produces pushback—so I think it is important to offer and invite, but not demand, one visit. In our studies of SST, we have been careful to refer to the 'POSSIBILITY of one session being enough' and to say 'When the first session MAY be the last'.
>
> (Hoyt, 2018: 157)

The pluralistic mindset in SST

Given that there is no specific approach to SST, this way of working can incorporate seemingly different approaches. It can do this because of its pluralistic nature or what may be referred to as working with 'both/and' rather than with 'either/or'. In discussing his own work, Talmon (2018: 153) writes about working with opposite poles. For example:

- On one pole, to validate a patient's story via empathic listening and on the other pole to challenge the problematic elements in the same storyline.
- On one pole, to increase a sense of hope or a realistic sense of optimism, and on the other pole helping him/her to accept certain parts of the harsh reality.
- There is an essential balance between offering neutral (and at times passive, silent) listening in one part of a session, and in another part, presenting active, focused questions.
- Similarly, between being non-directive at one point of the session, while at other times giving prescriptive-like directions.

SST as a mode of service delivery

As we have seen, some people in the field consider that SST is best viewed as a mode of service delivery and not an approach to delivering such services. As a service delivery mode, it utilises time in a very efficient way. Therapy is made available quickly and the time spent in therapy is kept as short as possible according to what the client wants.

The goals of SST

What can be realistically achieved by clients from SST? The following are examples of goals (Dryden, 2019b):

- to help the client get 'unstuck'
- to help the client take a few steps forward which may help them to travel the rest of the journey without professional assistance
- to help the client see that they have the wherewithal to achieve their goals

- to help the client select a possible solution to their problem
- to give the client the experience of the solution, if possible
- to help the client develop an action plan.

If clients have goals that are unrealistic in terms of what they can usefully achieve from SST, then their therapists should explain why this may be the case and attempt to set more realistic goals. If this can't be done, then SST should not be initiated (Dryden, 2019b).

Who is suitable for SST?

Whenever I give a talk on SST, it is inevitable that I will be asked a question concerning for whom and for which problems it is indicated and not indicated. When I first became interested in SST and developed my own private practice-based approach, I outlined a long list of indications and contraindications for this way of working (Dryden, 2017). While on the one hand this approach makes sense, on the other hand it raises the issue of carrying out a suitability-based assessment before therapy is initiated. As I showed earlier in this article in Table 1.1, one of the features of help provided at the point of need is that therapy begins at the very first moment of the therapy session. Given this, I modified my approach, and when a client contacts me, I outline the range of services that I offer, including SST, and invite the client to choose in the first instance if SST is something they think they can utilise. If so, I initiate SST and suggest a different service if it becomes clear that the client would do better with this other service. This latter decision is a jointly taken one.

The main objection to using suitability-based criteria comes from SST as practised in 'walk-in' settings. A client who seeks help from a walk-in clinic knows that they will be seen quickly and that this may be the only session that they have. They know that it is not the first session of a series of sessions stretching into the future. The therapist will see the client without knowing anything about them, the nature of their problem or what help they are seeking. The fact that the therapist is prepared to see the client under such conditions suggests that suitability-based assessment is not necessary and some would say not even desirable as it would represent a barrier between help sought and help offered.

Young (2018: 44) argued that the best response to the 'who is suitable?' question is to avoid having to answer it by embedding SST in the service system so that clients can return if they want to. Embedding SST into the service system so that all services the organization normally provides are available following an initial session, conducted as if it may be the last, allows the practitioner and the organization to avoid the 'difficult if not impossible' decision of who is suitable and who is not suitable for a 'one-off' session.

Additionally, as noted earlier, determining who will attend once and who will attend further sessions is a difficult enterprise and one that clinicians are not particularly good at.

SST occurs in a context

Before I discuss the practice of SST in detail, I want to make the point that this practice takes place in a context which needs to be understood. Talmon (2018: 150–151) notes that a

> one-at-a-time approach is embraced successfully where the need is much larger than the supply and where the therapists are working as a team with training and research being an active part of the process, and where the therapist's income is not based on a fee-for-time nor based on the assumption that more is always better.

However, when SST has been introduced into an agency by one or two enthusiasts who are not supported by most practitioners working in that environment, and with administrative support at a minimum, then it will not flourish in the agency. Please bear this in mind while reading about the practice of SST.[4]

Good practice in SST

A number of people in the SST field have put forward suggestions about what constitutes good practice in SST (e.g. Bloom, 1981, 1992; Dryden, 2019b; Hoyt, Rosenbaum, & Talmon, 1992; Slive & Bobele, 2011; Talmon, 1990, 1993). Table 1.2 outlines many of these suggestions for good practice in SST.

Table 1.2 **Elements of good practice in SST**

The effective single-session therapist:

- *engages the client as quickly as possible*
- *develops rapport through the work*
- *takes their time.* The therapist and the client have sufficient time to achieve something useful in the session.
- *encourages the client to understand the nature of SST, what is possible and what is not, and to choose whether or not they want SST*
- *is overt and collaborative with the client when deciding how much therapeutic contact is required*
- *is client-centred.* Clients are experts in reporting what kind of and how much change is important for them at any particular time. So, the therapist needs to focus on what the client wants.
- *speaks clearly and at a rate which maximises the client's participation and understanding*
- *whenever practicable, explains what they are doing.* However, it is important that they are not obsessive about doing so.
- *asks and explores what the client wants from the* <u>session</u> *rather than from* <u>therapy</u>. In doing so, they are fully aware that therapy may last for only one session.
- *is active-directive while encouraging the client's active participation in the process*
- *is focused and helps the client stay focused*
- *interrupts the client to preserve the session focus once negotiated when necessary.* The therapist should give a prior rationale for doing this and elicit the client's agreement. When interrupting, the effective therapist does so with tact.
- *keeps checking that they and the client are on the right track.* Thus, the therapist should shift the agenda to meet the client's concerns.
- *adopts a solution-oriented stance but, when necessary, is problem-focused.* Many SST therapists practice solution-focused therapy where the focus is on 'solution talk' and not 'problem talk' (Furman & Ahola, 1992). However, as we have seen, SST is practised by therapists from diverse orientations and in some a focus on problems is deemed helpful in SST. So, while it is difficult to think of SST that is not solution-oriented, the therapist should feel free also to focus on problems if this helps the selection of suitable solutions.

  [The next two items are relevant for SST therapists who deal with client problems.]

- *elicits the problem from the client's perspective*

***Table 1.2* Cont.**

- *assesses the problem*
- *elicits the client's goal/preferred future and keeps focused on this*
- *ensures that this forward focus is underpinned by a value if possible*
- *asks what the client is prepared to sacrifice to achieve the goal/preferred future*
- *bridges to the future whenever possible*
- *encourages the client to be as specific as possible but be mindful of opportunities for generalisation*
- *makes liberal use of questions*
- *ensures that the client answers the questions they are asked*
- *gives the client time to answer questions.* The therapist should remember that they have more time than they may think.
- *checks out the client's understanding of and reaction to substantive points that they have made to the client*
- *identifies and responds to the client's doubts, reservations and objections, including those that may be expressed non-verbally*
- *identifies and makes use of the client's strengths*
- *identifies the client's previous attempts to solve the problem.* The therapist should capitalise on the client's successful attempts and distance themself from the client's unsuccessful attempts.
- *identifies and utilises the client's learning style, if possible*
- *identifies and makes use of the external resources available to the client.* Factors external to therapy can be as important as those internal to therapy and sometimes more so.
- *looks for ways of making an emotional impact.* However, they should not push to bring about an emotional response.
- *encourages the client to take at least one meaningful point from the session and to have a plan to implement this point*
- *helps the client to select a possible solution to their problem that makes most sense to them and fits their life situation*
- *encourages the client to practise the solution in the session if possible*
- *helps the client to plan to implement the solution in their everyday life and encourages them to determine how this goes before they seek additional help*
- *encourages the client to summarise the session and they should themself add any missing points*
- *ties up any loose ends*
- *agrees criteria for further sessions with the client*
- *plans for a follow-up with the client*

What to avoid doing in SST

There are a number of practices that, while useful in certain situations, are generally to be avoided in SST. Other practices are generally not useful in therapy, but the time-sensitive nature of SST means that some therapists may be prone to use them. Practices to avoid in SST are outlined in Table 1.3.

Getting SST off on the right foot

When SST is practised in walk-in clinics, the therapist and client need to get down to work immediately. However, when SST is by appointment, the therapeutic dyad has an opportunity to do some preparatory work to get the process off on the right foot before they meet. I discuss one approach to this which is an example of what Hoyt (2000, 2018) refers to as the pre-session phase of SST where induction and seeding occur.

An example of a pre-session questionnaire

I designed a questionnaire which I use to inform a pre-session telephone contact that I have with a client. This takes place a day or two before the session itself (Dryden, 2017). Here are the questions that I ask:

- What is the one problem or concern that seems most important to focus on now?
- How does this problem affect: i) You?; ii) Other people in your life?
- What would be important for me to know about the background of this problem?
- What have you tried that has helped you with this problem?
- What have you tried that has not helped with the problem or made it worse?
- What would you like to get out of the session when we meet?
- How will you know when you have achieved the changes you desire?
- Remember a problem that happened any time in your life that you resolved in such a way that left you feeling proud of yourself. What did you do that you felt proud of?

Table 1.3 **Practices to avoid in SST**

• *The therapist should not* take an elaborate history.* If the therapist does so, this may take up the entire session and they won't have time to do any therapeutic work with the client.
• *The therapist should not let the client talk in an unfocused, general way.* While certain clients may gain benefit from a single session of unfocused exploration, most won't.
• *The therapist should not spend too much time in non-directive, listening mode.* The exception to this is when a client says that the best way the therapist can help them is just to listen.
• *The therapist should not develop rapport independent of the task of SST.* In SST, showing a client that the therapist is keen to help them as quickly as possible is perhaps the best way to strengthen the therapeutic bond.
• *The therapist should not assess where not relevant.* When the therapist assesses the client's problem, the assessment should stay focused on the problem.
• *The therapist should not carry out an elaborate case conceptualisation.* There is not sufficient time in SST for such a conceptualisation to be done. This poses a difficulty for CBT therapists who hold that therapy needs to be conceptualisation-driven.
• *The therapist should not assume that the client knows what the therapist is doing or why they are doing it.* Explicitness and clarity are hallmarks of good SST.
• *The therapist should not rush the client.*
• *The therapist should not ask multiple questions.* This is a specific sign that the therapist is rushing.
• *The therapist should not leave the client hanging at the end of the session.* Session closure is important.

* In this table, I use the term 'should not' to mean 'ideally should not'.

- What strengths as a person do you have that could help you deal with the problem effectively? What would people who know you really well say in answer to the same question?
- Who in your life right now could support you as you address the problem?
- For me to be most helpful to you, is there anything you feel it is vital for me to know about your culture, ethnicity, religion,

language, sexual orientation, gender identity/expression, mental or physical health, or other?

- What questions would you like addressed in the session?[5]

Not all of the above information is used in the single session, of course. However, it is there for the therapist and client to make use of, if needed. Sometimes this pre-session telephone contact is in itself sufficient to help the person consider that they can deal with their problem without further therapeutic contact.

In addition to these questions, the therapist might suggest a task that the client can do before the face-to-face session to initiate the process of change.

An example of the structure of a single session

You may be wondering what the structure of a single session looks like. In what follows, I present an example of such a structure as it is used by a university counselling service in the United Kingdom. Before attending, the client knows that the service is run on OAATT lines. This means that while the therapist will try to help them deal with the problem in the session, further sessions are available, but may be booked only one at a time.

- The therapist begins by explaining the service and the amount of time that the client has with them.
- The therapist explains the service's confidentiality policy and refers the client to its written policy statement if they require more detailed information.
- The therapist asks, 'What is the single most important concern that you have right now?'
- The therapist and client explore the most important type of help needed.
- The therapeutic dyad prioritises the client's needs. The therapist keeps the client's most immediate and critical needs a priority, yet is still mindful of their other needs.
- The therapist assesses if the client is at risk (suicide/self-harm or harm to others) and takes appropriate action.
- The therapist asks, 'People usually try to resolve a problem themselves. What things have you tried?'
- The therapist encourages the client to continue to use strategies that they have found helpful and discourages the future use of unhelpful strategies.

- The therapist asks, 'What inner strengths and resiliency factors do you have that it would it be useful for me to know about that might help you deal with the problem?' If necessary, the therapist educates the client about key strengths and resiliency factors (e.g., strong family relationships and friendships, positive outlook, spiritual convictions, sense of hope, feelings of personal control, creativity, persistence and humour). The therapist explains the role of inner strengths and resiliency factors as crucial components of the process of moving forward.
- The therapist asks, 'What external resources can you make use of in dealing with your prioritised concern?' The therapist asks in particular about people who may support the client through the change process and relevant agencies that may provide help.
- The therapist then asks, 'What would be the smallest change needed to show you that things are heading in the right direction?'
- It is here that the therapist searches for a solution, which may include offering approach-based insights as well as what the client thinks will be helpful.[6]
- Once a possible solution has been agreed upon, the therapist encourages the client to practise the solution in the session.
- The therapist helps the client to develop an action plan, perhaps negotiating a specific task to initiate the change process.
- The therapist encourages the client to ask any questions, which are answered before bringing the session to a close. In particular, the therapist might ask a question such as: 'What question(s) will you wish you had asked me when you get home today?'
- Finally, the therapist draws the client's attention to resources in the service's resource material or to 'apps' as appropriate.
- If the client expresses a wish to book a further session, the therapist encourages them first to reflect on what they have learned, digest it, take appropriate action and let time pass. However, the therapist reminds the client that a further session is possible with themself or with another counsellor.
- Finally, appropriate follow-up and evaluation are organised.

Misconceptions about SST

As noted by Jeff Young (2018), the term 'single-session therapy' is something of a misnomer which should be retained because it serves as a catalyst for important debates about service delivery and what clients actually want from therapy as opposed to what clinicians think they should have. However, there are terms that therapists new to this field often have misconceptions about (Weir et al., 2008; Young, 2018). In this final section, I will detail some of these misconceptions and put the record straight.

SST is a model of therapy in itself

As I argued earlier, SST is best seen as a mindset or an attitude towards clinical work or a mode of service delivery. It is not a discrete therapy model or therapeutic approach.

SST is the answer to everything

As Young (2018) has noted, SST is a mode of service delivery that stands with other modes of service delivery. Thus, at the Bouverie Centre in Melbourne, Australia, where Young is Director, all new clients have a single session and then decisions are made collaboratively about what further therapy the client needs, if any. Here, SST is seen as an entry hub. It is definitely not seen as the answer to all clinical problems

SST is a quick fix

The Cambridge dictionary online defines a quick fix as 'something that seems to be a fast and easy solution but is, in fact, not very good or will not last very long'. As discussed in the section on the goals of SST, the purpose of this mode of service delivery is to help the person get unstuck or take a few steps towards their goal. In addition, it helps the person to see that they have internal strengths and external resources on which they can call to address their problem. In OAATT, in particular, a client is encouraged to try out an agreed solution to a problem and see what transpires and to make another appointment if further help is needed. This is far from a 'quick fix'.

SST is better than other modes of service delivery because it saves money

While it is probably the case that SST as a mode of service delivery is cheaper to run than other modes such as time-limited or ongoing therapy, this is not a sound clinical rationale for its employment. As already mentioned, SST is best seen as a way of approaching clinical work that stands alongside and may feed into other delivery modes. It does not deem to compete with these other modes. Additionally, it is the intention of SST proponents to provide what clients most want, rather than trying to save money. It just happens to be the case that when practitioners focus on what clients want, doing so tends to shorten therapy and hence save money.

SST means a restriction on the therapy sessions

If a therapy agency has sufficient resources to offer all clients what they require, there would be no need to restrict services. However, even under these circumstances, it is clear from the data that many clients will still choose to only attend one, two or three sessions (Hoyt & Talmon, 2014b; Young, 2018). So, even when there is not a reason to restrict the number of therapy sessions, most clients will still choose to attend very briefly. The main point here is that the provision of SST does not and should not mean that certain clients should not receive more help if they need it and want it. And when they do receive such help, SST training helps practitioners be more client focused during longer-term work.

SST means one session

As I have already discussed, while there are some people in the SST field who apply the 'Ronseal' definition of SST where single-session therapy means one session, and that is that, most people in the field recognise that SST does not preclude further sessions. For example, Cummings (1990) notes that single-session therapy is a good example of intermittent therapy through the life cycle where a client may have a series of single sessions at various key points in their life. In addition, one-at-a-time (OAATT) therapy may involve one session but does not preclude further sessions, albeit held one at a time.

SST is five, ten or more sessions 'distilled' into one

This criticism of SST implies a speeded-up approach to therapy where the therapist crams a great deal of work into a single session. While a single session of therapy does have its own beginning, middle and ending phases (Hoyt, 2018), this process takes full account of the integrity of the single session that is being conducted and does not seek to condense much longer therapy into one therapy session. You can only do one session in one session.[7]

SST is the same as crisis intervention

While SST is an appropriate mode of service delivery for clients in crisis, it is not equivalent to crisis intervention. It can be and is used for clients who are in crisis and indeed can often help clients stave off such crises.

SST is simpler than longer-term therapy because it is brief and focused

Actually, the converse may be the case. SST requires the therapist to have well-developed therapeutic skills and thus may be more complex to practise than longer-term therapy.

SST is for everyone

While anyone may turn up at a walk-in clinic, that does not mean that SST is for everyone. As already discussed, a single session may be given to all who seek help at a clinic, and if a more appropriate service is indicated, then a jointly agreed referral is made. At the Bouverie centre in Melbourne, Australia, everyone gets a single session, and further work, if needed, is provided by the same therapist, not referred out. Young (personal communication, 12/1/19) states that 'longer term work is part of the outcomes of an initial session conducted using the SST service delivery approach. For example, in our service, our initial research showed 50% of SST clients decided on attending only 1 session, 25% a further "single session" and 24% ongoing work, all of which was provided by the same therapist.'

SST is only suitable for clients facing simple problems

Given that clients with a range of problems from the simple to the complex have sought help from and benefited from SST, this criticism comes more from therapists than from clients or service users. The latter have shown a high degree of satisfaction with the SST services that they have received (Hoyt & Talmon, 2014b; Hoyt et al., 2018a).

In this chapter, I have attempted to review the nature and current status of SST. In the following chapters, I explore the possible future of SST by interviewing three of the world's leaders in this field: Moshe Talmon from Israel, Michael Hoyt from the USA, and Jeff Young from Australia.[8] I asked them three questions:

- What are your predictions for the future of SST (i.e. what do you think will happen)?
- What are your hopes for the future of SST?
- What are your fears concerning the future of SST?

Notes

1 As seen by the author. In this chapter I will use the term 'single-session therapy' to also stand for 'One-At-A-Time Therapy' (OAATT) and will only use the latter term when it is pertinent to do so.
2 'IAPT' stands for 'Improving Access to Psychological Therapies'. Increasingly, people in Britain are contacting their local IAPT service for help directly rather than going to their GP, thereby reducing some waiting time. However, there still remains a significant waiting period and my main point holds.
3 In 1994, a British company called 'Ronseal' that manufactures wood stain, paint and preservatives developed a slogan to explain and demystify its products: 'Ronseal. It does exactly what it says on the tin.' This caught the public imagination to the extent that the phrase is used internationally and is now a commonly used slogan.
4 See Weir et al. (2008) for suggestions on how to implement SST into a service.
5 This question is asked by therapists working at the Bouverie Centre in Melbourne, Australia (Young, personal communication, 7/1/19).
6 In family therapy based on SST lines, in addition to the therapist or therapist team there may be observers present who, during a planned break in the therapy action, suggest possible solutions for the client and therapist(s) to consider when the action is resumed.
7 A point attributed to Robert Rosenbaum (Young, personal communication, 12/1/19).
8 I would like to thank Michael Hoyt, Moshe Talmon and Jeff Young for the generous gift of their time in agreeing to be interviewed and for reviewing the transcripts of the interviews.

References

Appelbaum, S.A. (1975). Parkinson's Law in psychotherapy. *International Journal of Psychoanalytic Psychotherapy, 4*, 426–436.

Bloom, B.L. (1981). Focused single-session therapy: Initial development and evaluation. In S. Budman (Ed.), *Forms of Brief Therapy* (pp. 167–216). New York: Guilford Press.

Bloom, B.L. (1992). *Planned Short-Term Psychotherapy: A Clinical Handbook*. Boston, MA: Allyn and Bacon.

Bloom, B.L. (2001). Focused single session psychotherapy: A review of the clinical and research literature. *Brief Treatment and Crisis Intervention, 1*(1), 75–86.

Campbell, A. (2012). Single-session approaches to therapy: Time to review. *Australian and New Zealand Journal of Family Therapy, 33*(1), 15–26.

Cummings, N.A. (1990). Brief intermittent psychotherapy through the life cycle. In J.K. Zeig & S.G. Gilligan (Eds.), *Brief Therapy: Myths, Methods and Metaphors* (pp. 169–194). New York: Brunner/Mazel.

Dryden, W. (2017). *Single-Session Integrated CBT (SSI-CBT): Distinctive Features*. Abingdon, Oxon: Routledge.

Dryden, W. (2019a). *Single-Session 'One-At-A-Time Therapy': A Rational Emotive Behaviour Therapy Approach*. Abingdon, Oxon: Routledge.

Dryden, W. (2019b). *Single-Session Therapy: 100 Key Points and Techniques*. Abingdon, Oxon: Routledge.

Freud, S., & Breuer, J. (1895). *Studien über Hysterie*. Leipzig and Vienna: Deuticke.

Furman, B., & Ahola, T. (1992). *Solution Talk: Hosting Therapeutic Conversations*. New York: Norton.

Hoyt, M.F. (2000). *Some stories are better than others: Doing what works in brief therapy and managed care*. Philadelphia, PA: Brunner/Mazel.

Hoyt, M.F. (2011). Foreword. In A. Slive & M. Bobele (Eds.), *When One Hour Is All You Have: Effective Therapy for Walk-In Clients* (pp. xix–xv). Phoenix, AZ: Zeig, Tucker, & Theisen.

Hoyt, M.F. (2018). Single-session therapy: Stories, structures, themes, cautions, and prospects. In M.F. Hoyt, M. Bobele, A. Slive, J. Young, & M. Talmon (Eds.), *Single-Session Therapy by Walk-In or Appointment: Administrative, Clinical, and Supervisory Aspects of One-at-a-Time Services* (pp. 155–174). New York: Routledge.

Hoyt, M.F., Bobele, M., Slive, A., Young, J., & Talmon, M. (2018a). Introduction: One-at-a-time/single-session walk-in therapy. In M.F. Hoyt, M. Bobele, A. Slive, J. Young, & M. Talmon (Eds.), *Single-Session Therapy by Walk-In or Appointment: Administrative, Clinical, and Supervisory Aspects of One-at-a-Time Services* (pp. 3–24). New York: Routledge.

Hoyt, M.F., Bobele, M., Slive, A., Young, J., & Talmon, M. (Eds.) (2018b). *Single-Session Therapy by Walk-In or Appointment: Administrative, Clinical, and Supervisory Aspects of One-at-a Time Services*. New York: Routledge.

Hoyt, M.F., & Dryden, W. (2018). Toward the future of single-session therapy: An interview. *Journal of Systemic Therapies, 37*(1), 79–89.

Hoyt, M.F., Rosenbaum, R., & Talmon, M. (1992). Planned single-session psychotherapy. In S.H. Budman, M.F. Hoyt, & S. Friedman (Eds.), *The First Session in Brief Therapy* (pp. 59–86). New York: Guilford Press.

Hoyt, M.F., & Talmon, M.F. (2014a). (Eds.). *Capturing the Moment: Single Session Therapy and Walk-In Services*. Bethel, CT: Crown House Publishing.

Hoyt, M.F., & Talmon, M.F. (2014b). What the literature says: An annotated bibliography. In M.F. Hoyt & M. Talmon (Eds.), *Capturing the Moment: Single Session Therapy and Walk-In Services* (pp. 487–516). Bethel, CT: Crown House Publishing.

Hymmen, P., Stalker, C.A., & Cait, C.-A. (2013). The case for single-session therapy: Does the empirical evidence support the increased prevalence of this service delivery model? *Journal of Mental Health, 22*(1), 60–67.

Kuehn, J.L. (1965). Encounter at Leyden: Gustav Mahler consults Sigmund Freud. *Psychoanalytic Review, 52*, 345–364.

Lazarus, A.A. (1981). *The Practice of Multimodal Therapy.* New York: McGraw-Hill.

Slive, A., & Bobele, M. (Eds.) (2011). *When One Hour Is All You Have: Effective Therapy for Walk-In Clients.* Phoenix, AZ: Zeig, Tucker & Theisen.

Slive, A., & Bobele, M. (2014). Walk-in single-session therapy: Accessible mental health services. In M.F. Hoyt & M. Talmon (Eds.), *Capturing the Moment: Single Session Therapy and Walk-In Services* (pp. 73–94). Bethel, CT: Crown House Publishing.

Talmon, M. (1990). *Single Session Therapy: Maximizing the Effect of the First (and Often Only) Therapeutic Encounter.* San Francisco, CA: Jossey-Bass.

Talmon, M. (1993). *Single Session Solutions: A Guide to Practical, Effective and Affordable Therapy.* New York: Addison-Wesley.

Talmon, M. (2018). The eternal now: On becoming and being a single-session therapist. In M.F. Hoyt, M. Bobele, A. Slive, J. Young, & M. Talmon (Eds.), *Single-Session Therapy by Walk-In or Appointment: Administrative, Clinical, and Supervisory Aspects of One-at-a-Time Services* (pp. 149–154). New York: Routledge.

Weir, S., Wills, M., Young, J., & Perlesz, A. (2008). *The Implementation of Single Session Work in Community Health.* Brunswick, Victoria, Australia: The Bouverie Centre, La Trobe University.

Young, J. (2018). SST: The misunderstood gift that keeps on giving. In M.F. Hoyt, M. Bobele, A. Slive, J. Young, & M. Talmon (Eds.), *Single-Session Therapy by Walk-In or Appointment: Administrative, Clinical, and Supervisory Aspects of One-at-a-Time Services* (pp. 40–58). New York: Routledge.

Chapter 2

The future of single-session therapy

An interview with Moshe Talmon[1]

Introduction

One of the first therapists who practised single-session therapy (SST) was Sigmund Freud. It is reported that the pioneer of long-term psychoanalysis carried out two well-known single-session treatments, one with Aurelia Öhm-Kronich ('Katharina') in 1893 (Freud & Breuer, 1895) and the other with the famous composer Gustav Mahler in 1910 (Kuehn, 1965). While there are periodic references to single-session treatment in the literature from that time onwards, with well-known therapists like Alfred Adler, Milton Erickson and Albert Ellis pioneering the use of single therapy sessions often conducted in front of professional and lay audiences, it wasn't until 1990 that the field of SST began to cohere. This is when Moshe Talmon, the subject of the following interview, published a book which many, including myself, consider seminal and which marked the beginning of a growing interest in SST by appointment or by walk-in.

In the 1980s, Talmon left a comfortable private therapy practice in Israel to work at the world renowned public Kaiser Permanente clinic in Oakland, California. He discovered for the first time in his professional life that many patients that he saw in the clinic only attended for one session. He wondered whether he had suddenly become a bad therapist with lots of 'drop-outs' to his name. While his professional pride was bruised, his curiosity was stronger and he took the step of telephoning 200 of his one-session patients to find that many of them had been very satisfied with their session and did not feel the need for continuing therapy. From those early pioneering days, SST has challenged commonly held ideas such as that psychological change occurs gradually and that treatment should only be initiated after a thorough case formulation has been undertaken.

One of the intriguing aspects of single-session therapy is that it is not necessarily therapy that lasts for one session and that is it. Rather, it is a way of approaching therapy where therapist and client work together to see if they can help the latter get what they want from one session, but, if not, more help is available. Paradoxically, it is knowing that more help is possible that enables the client to relax and get the most from *the first and often only therapeutic encounter.*[2]

Against this backdrop, I interviewed Moshe Talmon about his views on the future of SST.

> **Windy:** What do you think have been the key developments in single-session therapy since 1990?
>
> **Moshe:** Well, there was quite a bit that happened since the publication of my first book in 1990. One development that was surprising to me was that, when we started the series of the SST studies at Kaiser Permanente Medical Group in 1986, we assumed that single-session therapy would suit mostly the so-called 'worried well' and maybe a few of the adjustment disorders.
>
> Since the publication of the book (Talmon, 1990), both during training that I was invited to do all over the world and the research and publications done by other people around the world, it appears that single-session therapy can help people with much more complex and difficult problems than I originally assumed.
>
> Initially, when people would call me to ask for training in SST, for example, those who were working with teenagers who live on the streets, with sexually and physically abused women, with cancer patients, with addicts of different kinds, etc. I would tell them that I know nothing about what can be done in a single session with people who clearly need much longer therapy, and they would keep telling me that this is the most common length of therapy with these clients, and therefore they would like to try and utilise single-session work with them.
>
> So that was a surprising development that I'm glad to say today challenged me and forced me to think in different ways about single-session therapy.

The second development is the development of walk-in clinics where single-session therapy is actually the main modality that is used in the clinic, and what more recently we called the 'one-at-a-time' model (Hoyt, Bobele, Slive, Young & Talmon, 2018). These clinics had a much higher frequency of single-session therapy than we did. In our study of planned SST (Talmon, 1990) it was 58% of the clients in our research sample, and in many of the walk-in clinics in Australia and Canada and the United States it is up to 80% of the clients. So that was a second development that was very interesting.

The third development is the use of single-session therapy in non-psychotherapy services – counselling services carried out by people who don't see themselves as psychotherapists; they see themselves as counsellors, they see themselves as coaches. In addition, I trained medical staff, primary care physicians family specialists and nurses in SST.

Windy: What are your predictions about how single-session therapy will develop in the future?

Moshe: Well, I know that you indicated, in your book, that you were interested in the future of single-session therapy, but in Hebrew we have a saying that I think you also know in English. It is that 'predictions are for fools'. So, I would prefer to talk about what are my hopes for the future of single-session therapy.

Windy: OK, so let's structure it according to your hopes and fears, shall we?

Moshe: Right. My first hope is that single-session therapy will be integrated with all services and with various approaches to therapy.

My second hope is that SST is utilised in what is called today 'advanced systems' such as the sharing economy and social media. In this way, everyone can help make therapy more accessible and more affordable, by combining, for example, artificial intelligence and social media. However, I think that, despite these technological developments, the importance of face-to-face interaction and human intuition, and the therapeutic alliance, in particular, is still very vital. So I hope that the developments in artificial intelligence and in big data will make therapy more accessible, but that this is combined with the use of the face-to-face human inter-action. So, both/and, not either/or.

My third hope is that while evidence-based therapy places a lot of importance on protocols, single-session therapy, while being evidence-based, will be individually tailored to each client rather than be protocol driven.

Windy: So it's important not to lose the human interaction, therapeutic alliance, sort of flesh and blood nature of the work.

Moshe: Exactly. There is always the fear that artificial intelligence will exclude the human touch, but I think that, especially in psychological terms, everything that helps to create a therapeutic alliance, such as emotional intelligence and social intelligence, are not going to be replaced by artificial intelligence; indeed, to the contrary.

Windy: So, before we go onto your fears, your third hope is for what my good friend Arnold Lazarus (1981) used to call 'the bespoke nature of psychotherapy' in that SST would be individually tailored and would not fall foul of this current drive to protocol everything. So, although there are guidelines, of course, to practise single-session therapy, the important thing is to utilise these guidelines and tailor them to the individual, rather than to fit the individual to the protocol.

Moshe: Right. I hope that we will be flexible enough and ver-satile enough to meet each client at their place and time.

Windy: What about your fears for the future development of SST?

Moshe: The main concern that I have is that powerful and big systems – be it governmental agencies, insurance com-panies or HMOs – will use the power and the effectiveness of single-session therapy to block access to populations that are in most need of psychotherapy. So, if single-session therapy is used, let's say, with poor people, single parents or people who live on the streets, and those controlling access to therapy say, 'OK, we will give you only one session, and you don't need more than that,' or, 'We will give you one indi-vidual session and then we will send you to group sessions,' then I think that it will be an abuse of single-session therapy. Is that clear?

Windy: Yes, and I agree with that entirely.

Moshe: And one more concern, which I expressed also in the last chapter that I wrote on the subject (Talmon, 2018), I think that we have to be concerned that people will not use our findings and our successes with single-session therapy to narrow or flatten human struggle and human suffering into 'one size fits all'. That can be done by some people and it should be avoided.

Windy: Yes, I agree with that. Thank you, Moshe, for your time.

Notes

1 Conducted on 19/02/18 and revised on 24/03/20.
2 This italicised phrase is taken from the subtitle of Talmon's (1990) book.

References

Freud, S., & Breuer, J. (1895). *Studien über Hysterie*. Leipzig and Vienna: Deuticke.

Hoyt, M.F., Bobele, M., Slive, A., Young, J., & Talmon, M. (Eds.) (2018). *Single-Session Therapy by Walk-In or Appointment: Administrative, Clinical, and Supervisory Aspects of One-at-a-Time Services*. New York: Routledge.

Kuehn, J.L. (1965). Encounter at Leyden: Gustav Mahler consults Sigmund Freud. *Psychoanalytic Review, 52*, 345–364.

Lazarus, A.A. (1981). *The Practice of Multimodal Therapy*. New York: McGraw-Hill.

Talmon, M. (1990). *Single Session Therapy: Maximizing the Effect of the First (and Often Only) Therapeutic Encounter*. San Francisco, CA: Jossey-Bass.

Talmon, M. (2018). The eternal now: On becoming and being a single-session therapist. In M.F. Hoyt, M. Bobele, A. Slive, J. Young, & M. Talmon (Eds.), *Single-Session Therapy by Walk-In or Appointment: Administrative, Clinical, and Supervisory Aspects of One-at-a-Time Services* (pp. 149–154). New York: Routledge.

Chapter 3

Toward the future of single-session therapy

An interview with Michael F. Hoyt

Overview

The possibilities of one-session therapy have been receiving increased attention since the publication of Moshe Talmon's best-selling 1990 book *Single Session Therapy: Maximizing the Effects of the First (and Often Only) Therapeutic Encounter*. Working with Michael Hoyt and Robert Rosenbaum, Talmon reported that many clients found a single session to be useful and sufficient for a range of problems. Since then, *Single Session Therapy* has been translated into many languages, and numerous investigators (see Hoyt & Talmon, 2014; Hoyt, Bobele, Slive, Young & Talmon, 2018) have confirmed and extended the finding that one session can be, for many clients, all that they need.

The following interview with one of the originators and one of the adapters of the single-session therapy (SST) approach took place (via Skype, between London, England, and Mill Valley, California) on 2 February 2018.[1]

> **Windy:** So I thought I'd start with your view of where we are in single-session therapy from 1990. I dated it with the publication of Moshe's book. I am curious to see what your views are of what the key developments have been from 1990 up until now.
>
> **Michael:** I think there have been several developments since 1990. The first, I think, is the *much greater recognition of the prevalence or frequency* of single-session or one-session therapies. Prior to Moshe's book, there were scattered reports here and there, where you'd catch a clinical case, but as we have pulled together the literature it has become more

apparent that there are many of these reports. Quantitative utilization studies have also repeatedly demonstrated that one session is the most common length of treatment. So, one development is increased awareness of frequency.

A second, I think, is that there has been *much more research documenting the effectiveness* of one-session therapies. There have been a number of reviews, and we catalogued some of the studies in *Capturing the Moment* (Hoyt & Talmon, 2014). That's a second development since 1990.

A third development is that there has been recognition that different models – solution-focused, cognitive-behavioral, MRI, narrative, even psychodynamic – all can be helpful. So, we are beginning to see that *there is not just one way to do it.*

A different kind of important development has been the recognition that single-session therapy is not a particular theoretical approach, but rather *SST is a format or a delivery system*; the one-at-a-time idea that Arnie Slive and Monte Bobele (2011, 2018) especially have talked a lot about. So "single session" doesn't mean solution-focused therapy or CBT, etc., it really means "I'm going to help them today," approaching the session with the mind-set that this is a one-shot, a one-chance, let's-see-what-we-can-get-done-in-this-meeting opportunity. One-at-a-time doesn't necessarily mean there will be only one time, but each session is approached as complete unto itself. More sessions can be scheduled, if needed, but "single session" is really "this is it" rather than "we planned to keep meeting but stopped after one."

Those are some of the main developments. We are also hearing more and more that a single-session therapy was *effective with difficult cases*: drug abuse, domestic violence, suicide ideation, not just simple problems with living or easy adjustment disorders. That is where I have seen the field going since 1990.

Another piece to put in here is the idea that SST has become *much more international*. Moshe was here in the U.S. for a number of years, but he is Israeli. Bob Rosenbaum and I are Americans. We've all taught on several continents. Monte Bobele and Arnie Slive are also Americans, although Arnie lived for many years in Canada and helped found the walk-in clinic at Eastside Family Centre in Calgary (see Slive et al., 1995; Slive et al., 2008). To name just a few others: you are doing things in Britain and have been teaching your form of Single-Session Integrated CBT (SSI-CBT; Dryden, 2016, 2017, 2018) in places as far flung as Brazil and Dubai. There are also SST trainings in Italy; there is another group in Sweden; there is Jeff Young et al. doing great stuff in Australia; Bobele and Slive are doing excellent work with SST and walk-in clinics in Texas and in Mexico; Chris Iveson, Harvey Ratner, and Evan George are busy at BRIEF in London and around the world; Karen Young and Jim Duval and other people are teaching and doing fine work using narrative therapy walk-in SSTs in Canada and the U.S. Indeed, there has been an explosion of SST and walk-in clinics throughout the Province of Ontario since the recommendations of the policy paper *No More, No Less: Brief Mental Health Services for Children and Youth* (Duvall, Young, & Kayes-Burden, 2012; also see Young, 2018). So, it is becoming more internationally recognized. That is another development. In *Capturing the Moment* Moshe wrote about this: who would have ever thought, when we did our first little study with 58 subjects in 1990, in a suburb of San Francisco called Hayward, California, that we'd be talking with people in England and Italy and Sweden and everywhere else around the world. So that is quite a development.

Windy: Yes, from little acorns.

Michael: Indeed, from little acorns.

Windy: What I'm wanting to capture here is the distinction between what you predict is going to happen, what you hope will happen and what you fear might happen. I don't know if you are prepared to talk about all three of those issues.

Michael: I'll try. The American writer Mark Twain once said he never liked to make predictions, especially about the future. "The future" always depends on so many factors – the government, the economy, science, and everything else. The further we look into the future, it's harder to know. But I would predict there is going to be *more single-session therapy* – that's an obvious thing to say – and I think there are going to be *more walk-ins particularly*. Clinics are going to be more and more recognizing, "This is a very useful thing. We ought to have somebody sitting here so that anyone can walk in or call in, same-day service, same-day counselling." So, I think there's going to be more walk-ins.

A second prediction is that there is going to be *more Internet single-session therapy*; people using Skype, Facetime, WhatsApp or some another app, exchanging questions and answers or getting information online.[2] People doing therapy over the Internet has a whole series of issues, some having to do with jurisdiction and licensing. If I'm in California and doing therapy (SST or otherwise) with somebody in Rome, and they tell me something dangerous that worries me, do I report it to my local police or do I call the Roman police and report it? In addition to questions about jurisdictions and licensing, what are the standards in different places, who has responsibility for what? Even within the U.S., the rules are different state to state. There will be more Internet therapy, so these issues will need to get sorted out.

Windy: So that was your second prediction: there will be more Internet usage.

Michael: Yes. I also think there are going to be *more publications, more writing, more training, more teaching.*

How would I hope to see single-session develop? In several ways. I would like to see it develop that there are *clinics available everywhere*. It will be something people just know about: if you have a problem, you can call this number and go to this storefront, or you can go to this clinic and just walk in, that idea. There is especially a big need for more services for disadvantaged people, folks that can't afford so-called regular therapy, where you make an appointment every week and go and chat. This could be something, whether through the government and public support, or done privately, where agencies could get very involved in offering easily accessible mental-health services.

We recently had yet another round of terrible shootings in the United States, and there is a big hue and cry right now that we need more mental-health services. I'm not saying single-session therapy is the answer to the gun problem, but if there was something available that said, "Depressed? Thinking of harming yourself? There's somebody to call and help is waiting," that would be good.

Occasionally, when I'm driving my car, I will listen to some sports radio programs for a few minutes, and one of the sports radio fellows regularly has announcements about "Mental health is good for you, and, if you're hurting or feeling lonely, you should see somebody." It would be nice if there was a billboard that said, "1–800, call Windy," or "Call Michael," or something.

Another SST development that I would like to see is *much more attention to cultural nuances*; how you do therapy with Mexicans may be somewhat different than how you do it with Brits than how you do it with Swedes and how you do it with Australians or Chinese or people from the U.S. We need more appreciation of the different strengths in different cultures, how they go about it, valuing the different belief systems people are coming from. As Terry Soo-Hoo (2018) has written, therapy can be much more effective and efficient if you work within someone's cultural context, and it is especially important not to work against their culture. We're getting more aware of the importance of multiculturalism and diversity, but we've got a long way yet to go. I hope that we're going to see much more attention to how to work with different populations.

A further development that I would like to see is related to the next paper I've been thinking I would write about single-session therapy. I will probably call it "The Joy of SST." I'm very interested in approaches that elevate people's abilities, that see their strengths, that celebrate resources, capacities, the attitude of "Yes, I can" (see Hoyt, 2017). So I hope we're going to see *more developments that bring forward people's abilities*: "Maybe with a little help I can make a change," rather than, "I'm so screwed up and I'm so damaged, I'm just ruined." So, I'm hoping to see more elevation of strengths.

I do believe that diagnosis has a useful purpose at times; it points out where there are problems or weaknesses. But I think we've become terribly obsessed with diagnosis, dysfunction, and disease. The psychologist Kenneth Gergen (1994; also see Gergen, 2006) wrote a paper called "Therapeutic Professions and the Diffusion of Deficit" in which he discusses how we've spread pathologizing to everyone. We may sometimes have problems, but the often really destructive underlying message is: "I'm not OK, you're not OK, we're all really screwed-up wrecks." In an interview I did (Hoyt, 1994/2001) with Steve de Shazer and John Weakland, they noted that most therapists tend to function as mental-*illness* not mental-*health* professionals. Solution-focused, narrative, and other single-session work is usually more strengths-oriented or strengths-based; what's right and what people *can* do rather than what's broken and what they *can't* do.

What developments would I <u>not</u> like to see? I have a couple of ideas. I'm not sure how it gets paid for in different places, but in the United States *I do not want insurance companies to limit people to one session.* They could try to say, "Well, you know, they've got evidence now that one session helps a lot of people, so you can have one, and then, if that doesn't work, then you're not a candidate for therapy." Nick Cummings (2000) has cautioned about that. He said, "Single session can be right for some patients, but we should not interpret this too broadly."

I've seen a lot of clients that I helped in one visit and I've seen a lot of clients who needed a lot more than one visit – either they didn't have the internal wherewithal to pull it together or their external reality was just too much to deal with all at once, or their therapist didn't have enough skill to help them see the way through it quickly. Sometimes people need on-going support, they need longer-term help making changes. It becomes an interesting question in the theory of psychotherapy. In his foreword to *Single-Session Therapy*, Jerome Frank (1990) wrote about the idea of people making changes in one session of therapy violates or challenges a lot of the assumptions that therapists have had: the beliefs that you have to gradually form an alliance, you have to gradually uncover the underlying schemas or neuroses, you then have to gradually work your way through or there will be too much resistance. So, when things happen relatively quickly, it's an interesting challenge for researchers, what really happened, because it can't be a gradual working-through process; something shifted more quickly. So, another prediction would be *more research*, both on the processes that occur in single-session therapies as well as on the prevalence and cost-effectiveness of SST. Consistent with Jay Haley's (see Talmon, 1993, flyleaf) statement that "Now it appears that therapy of a single interview could become the standard for estimating how long and how successful therapy should be," I expect that we'll be seeing more exploration of what problems can be effectively addressed in a single session.

Windy: Would you also say that you wouldn't want practitioners to limit themselves to just doing single-session work?

Michael: I would not want practitioners limited to SST for several reasons. If you say that they can only see a client one time, most practitioners will never listen to you again. You'll lose your audience. They need to make a living. It's hard to do only single sessions. I think it's a good thing for practitioners to be oriented to the idea of one-at-a-time: "Let's sit down today and see what we can get done." It may be enough that we don't need to meet again, but let's not decide that, the client and I, until the session has really been completed – "Do you think this has been enough for now? How will you use it? What are your next steps? Do you want to make an appointment now? Do you want to check in? You can always call."

I remember when Moshe's book came out in 1990 – 28 years ago now – and there was an article in a local newspaper about me, because I was one of the investigators. And I got several telephone calls from people. I was the "single-session wizard" and I was going to "cure" unbelievable problems: I was going to fix bad marriages, make delinquent children behave. And I would try to break it down and so I'd ask, "What would be one small step in that direction?" or, "What would be a first indication?" – all those kinds of questions you'd ask. And a couple of people got mad at me for not having instant answers, and they said, "No, we were told you did one session therapy and solved problems." I said, "Well, I don't solve them. I help you solve them. You know how to eat an elephant? One bite at a time," etc., etc.

I think there will be a few practitioners who advertise themselves as single-session specialists or one-stop therapists, and I don't think that it's bad to say, "I do single session when we can, and I'm also available for intermittent or brief, and I'm also available for longer-term work. So, let's talk and sort it out." There are also walk-in clinics where people are on staff or are trainees, so that they have a salary and are not financially motivated to keep the same clients coming back over and over. Public recognition of the possibilities of SST is growing. There was an item in 2016 in the *Huffington Post*, and there is a cover story article (DeMelo, 2018) in *O: The Oprah Magazine* about single-session therapy.

Another thing *I would not want single session to become is a particular theoretical approach*; that it's only solution-focused, only cognitive-behavioral, or only strategic, or whatever. I think it's important to do what works for the particular client. It's good to have a model (or better yet, a couple of models), but it's also good to be eclectic in the sense you can draw from different approaches. Sometimes it's really helpful to talk about how a problem developed, sometimes it's really good to talk about when a problem isn't being a problem, sometimes it's good to teach a skill or even give advice. When I'm teaching a workshop on single-session therapy, someone will raise their hand and say, "So how do you do single-session therapy with bipolar manic patients?" or "How do you do single-session therapy with cutting borderlines?" As if there is one answer. I would not want to say there's only one approach. If we could get enough evidence, and if one approach really did seem to work better, then I might say, "Sure, the ideas and techniques of CBT seem to work well with anxiety disorders – how could those ideas fit with this particular person?" or, "DBT appears to be a good way to go with so-called borderlines – how can you and Mr. Jones adapt it for him?" If you're trying to resolve "Anxiety" or "Borderline-ism" I don't think it's going to be one session.

Windy: No, exactly. It depends upon what they want. I often say that people with borderline personality disorder also may have a particular problem with job interviews that they may need some help with.

Michael: Right. People who have schizophrenia also have this other condition called "life." I heard Jay Haley in a conference once, when somebody said, "I've got a borderline patient and they've got ADHD," Jay interrupted and said, "I would not let that be the problem. A problem is something you can have a solution to." There are these global indictments, "You're borderline," or, "You're manic," or, "You're whatever."

My experience is, people come in, maybe only once or twice, and almost no one (unless he or she is a therapist!) comes in and says, "I want to resolve my borderline personality disorder," or, "My narcissism needs taming." They come in saying, "I can't get a date," or, "I've got a sexual problem," or, "I'm always getting into a fight with my partner."

Windy: Exactly.

Michael: That's where the rubber meets the road.

Windy: So the two things you wouldn't like to see are the abuse of single-session therapy by insurance companies, limiting people to just one session; and you wouldn't like it to be just a particular approach across the board, although you're open to the possibility that research might show that specific approaches might be specifically helpful for specific problems.

Michael: Yes, you've paraphrased it very well. That's what I'm trying to say. Even though somebody will say, "My approach is solution-focused," or, "psychodynamic," or, "cognitive-behavioral," I still want to see what they really do with the clients, because there's this big global thing called "CBT," but they're doing a lot of things and maybe what's really making the difference is the supportive relationship. The research on common factors certainly suggests that the alliance and what the client brings are more important than the therapist's specific bag of techniques. So, we have to look at the nuts and bolts of the actual clinical interaction – the labels don't mean a lot anymore.

Windy: Just on that point, it just reminds me that I wrote two articles on a situation where Albert Ellis interviewed this woman, and, a few days later, I interviewed the woman on exactly the same problem (Dryden, 2010a, 2010b). It came out completely differently. So, labels don't tell you what you want to know.

Michael: That's a good example: two expert "REBT" practitioners using the same model and talking with the same client about the same problem, yet things came out completely differently. In SST (as in other therapies) we both "capture the moment" and "create the moment." "Schools" or labels don't really tell us much. They certainly don't have to be mutually exclusive, but I think "psychodynamic" is sometimes used to mean "I'm deep and profound," and "cognitive-behavioral" is used to mean "I'm clear and specific," and "strategic" is used to mean "I'm clever and trick people for their own good," and "solution-focused" is used to mean "I'm optimistic and up with people," and "narrative" is used to mean "I'm for the underdog and extra alert to the influence of language." I'm being a little facetious.

Windy: No, I understand.

Michael: On a good day, I try to be all of those. They have different theories and traditions, but then, when you ask, "What did you actually do?" you usually find that effective and efficient therapists have got a specific goal; they identified client strengths and resources, what the client could do differently (sometimes by looking at exceptions to the problem); they evoked hope and effort; and they encouraged and guided the client to use whatever had been successful before and also sometimes taught them new skills. The language and technologies may be different, but it seems like good practice comes together much more than these separate "theory silos" might suggest.

Windy: So are there any other developments you wouldn't like to see?

Michael: Those are the ones that come to mind right now. I have two questions, however, if I may, to ask back at you. Maybe now's not a good time, or maybe it is. I'm curious about your answers to the questions: "Are there other SST developments that you would not like to see?" and "What's your hope for the future of SST?"

Windy: Well, I wouldn't like to see the abuse of single-session therapy. Over here it's more like the National Health Service. There's a tension to be had between providing services when they're needed and just restricting people. So, I would like to see single-session work, particularly walk-in services, as you were saying before, offered here in Britain, with the National Health Service, but I think that, if that happened, then people who needed extra help might not be offered it. So, I think I would agree with that.

What I would hope to see is people trained more in the mind-set of single-session work. I'm very attracted to the idea that there's an SST mind-set that you can bring to on-going therapy. If you're seeing somebody in an on-going way, you could still have a single-session mind-set or a one-at-a-time mind-set. So, I'd like to see that kind of thing. I don't think people are well trained for that.

Michael: One session of therapy in a planned or expected on-going string is a different mind-set or orientation.

Windy: So I'd like to see people really trained to help people as quickly as possible. I'm a great believer in, a bit like after a meal, you digest things. So encouraging clients to have a session, and then not necessarily to make their mind up at the time, but to digest what they've learnt; to try it out and then to come back. I was always struck by Albert Ellis, because I've listened to many of his recordings, and, at the end of a session, he said, "OK, if you want to make another session, you can, by making an appointment at the front desk." So he would not make his own appointments, and he wouldn't say, "Go down and book a session," he would say, "If you want another session." So that's an interesting way of doing things, I think.

Michael: If I were coaching someone on how to build a long-term private practice of a few interminable patients, it would be the opposite of the single-session approach. Every session, at the end, I would have them say, "There are more things we need to talk about." I'd have them be very friendly as the session came to an end, "It's been so good seeing you, I look forward to our next time together." I would have them do all these things to make the clients feel they need to come back as opposed to conveying the message, "You've had a good meal, go home and digest it. In a week or two ring me up, tell me how it's settled and tell me if you want to come back for another." That's very different than that cycle of booking the next feeding while you're still having dessert.

Windy: I do a lot of demonstrations with people with, what I call, everyday problems of living; you've got a problem, you may talk it over with a friend, which is fine, but the friend may not be able to help you so much. There's a development in London where some people have got what I think they call the "Listening Booth." They've got it in various different parts of London, where you can pop in and talk to somebody for half-an-hour or so about something.

Michael: I've heard of that.

Windy: So, I'd like to see a lot more of that. I think I'd like to see things like offering second opinions and maybe having trainees experience different approaches to therapy, so that they can get, if you like, a taste of different therapies, not just read about them but experience them. So, it's quite a flexible perspective, I think.

Michael: Yes. The fact that SST can be thought of as a format rather than a particular approach, 60 minutes or 90 minutes is a chunk of time that allows a lot of variation within it, as opposed to "here's the six steps that you're to follow."

Windy: Exactly.

Michael: Another area of single session does have to do with *protocols and programs*, where people come and they're going to have a one-session experience where they participate in some kind of structured process. Psycho-educational health-psychology classes, like stress-reduction, stop-smoking, or improve-your-sleep, could fit here. There are also research-validated one-session treatments for specific phobias and nightmares (Davis III, Ollendick, & Öst, 2012). Numerous studies have shown that medical utilization is often reduced after one session of therapy, and a planned one session of motivational interviewing has also been shown repeatedly to be helpful with various problems (see Hoyt & Talmon, 2014; Hoyt et al., 2018).

There is also another kind of single session that Miller, Platt, and Conroy (2018) wrote about. They're working in Cambodia, sometimes with people who have been horribly damaged and disfigured by having had acid thrown in their faces, awful sorts of stuff. They organize a day that is a festival where all the survivors can dance and sing and be together, and feel again like human beings rather than being shunned and ostracized.

There may be, and I use the term loosely, indigenous or other cultural processes or ceremonies that offer a one-session healing experience. There are clients I have known who were very religious, and they said, "What was really helpful was when I went and prayed with Father Joseph," or, "when we had the ceremony at the synagogue" or "the ritual at the mosque," or wherever it was. So I think there's a possibility of "single session" sometimes losing the word "therapy" and gaining some other, non-stigmatized word. (This, of course, may affect what insurance will cover.) "Therapy" sounds very clinical; there is a psychological or psychiatric problem, a "mental disorder," that is "treated" in therapy. I don't know what the other word is exactly: "work" or "process" or "encounter" or "happening" – having some way of having an experience that's helpful and healing but not "clinical." There may be a problem that clinicians would recognize, but approaching it from a different perspective, whether it's social or cultural or spiritual-religious. The remedy might be something else, maybe an encounter with nature or art or theatre, or maybe even some smooth jazz.

Windy: Thank you so much for your time, Michael.

Michael: And thanks to you, too!

Notes

1 Some revisions to the transcript of this interview were made on 24/03/20.
2 As I write (24/03/20), most therapists in the world are currently doing therapy with their clients online due to the restrictions on face-to-face human contact stemming from the Coronavirus.

References

Cummings, N.A. (2000). The single session misunderstanding. In *The Collected Papers of Nicholas A. Cummings. Vol. 1: The Value of Psychological Treatment* (p. 77). Phoenix, AZ: Zeig, Tucker, & Theisen.

Davis III, T.E., Ollendick, T.H., & Öst, L.-G. (Eds.) (2012). *Intensive One-Session Treatment of Specific Phobias*. New York: Springer.

DeMelo, J. (2018, July). Bull's eye! One-and-done sessions give new meaning to the phrase targeted therapy. *O: The Oprah Magazine*, 63–64, 67.

Dryden, W. (2010a). Two REBT therapists and one client: Windy Dryden transcript. *Journal of Rational-Emotive and Cognitive-Behavior Therapy*, 28(3), 130–140.

Dryden, W. (2010b). Elegance in REBT: Reflections on the Ellis and Dryden sessions with Jane. *Journal of Rational-Emotive and Cognitive-Behavior Therapy*, 28(3), 157–163.

Dryden, W. (2016). *When Time Is at a Premium: Cognitive-Behavioural Approaches to Single-Session Therapy and Very Brief Coaching*. London: Rationality Publications.

Dryden, W. (2017). *Single-Session Integrated CBT (SSI-CBT)*. Abingdon, Oxon: Routledge.

Dryden, W. (2018). *Very Brief Therapeutic Conversations*. Abingdon, Oxon: Routledge.

Duvall, J., Young, K., & Kayes-Burden, A. (2012). *No More, No Less: Brief Mental Health Services for Children and Youth.* www.excellenceforchildandyouth.com

Frank, J.D. (1990). Foreword. In M. Talmon, *Single Session Therapy: Maximizing the Effect of the First (and Often Only) Therapeutic Encounter* (pp. xi-xiii). San Francisco, CA: Jossey-Bass.

Gergen, K.J. (1994). Therapeutic professions and the diffusion of deficit. In *Realities and Relationships: Soundings in Social Construction.* Cambridge. MA: Harvard University Press.

Gergen, K.J. (2006). Deficit discourse and cultural enfeeblement. In *Therapeutic Realities: Colloboration, Oppression and Relational Flow* (pp. 107–138). Chagrin Falls, OH: Taos Institute Publications.

Hoyt, M.F. (2001). On the importance of keeping it simple and taking the patient seriously: A conversation with Steve de Shazer and John Weakland. In M.F. Hoyt, *Interviews with Brief Therapy Experts* (pp. 1–33). New York: Brunner/Mazel [work originally published 1994].

Hoyt, M.F. (2017). *Brief Therapy and Beyond: Stories, Language, Love, Hope, and Time.* New York: Routledge.

Hoyt, M.F., Bobele, M., Slive, A., Young, J., & Talmon, M. (Eds.) (2018). *Single-Session Therapy by Walk-In or Appointment: Administrative, Clinical, and Supervisory Aspects of One-at-a-Time Services.* New York: Routledge.

Hoyt, M.F., & Talmon, M. (Eds.) (2014). *Capturing the Moment: Single Session Therapy and Walk-In Services.* Bethel, CT: Crown House Publishing.

Huffington Post (2016, August 30). Sometimes just one session of therapy can be enough. Retrieved online September 11, 2016.

Miller, J.K., Platt, J.J., & Conroy, K.M. (2018). Single-session therapy in the majority world: Addressing the challenge of service delivery in Cambodia and the implications for other global contexts. In M.F. Hoyt et al. (Eds.), *Single-Session Therapy by Walk-In or Appointment: Administrative, Clinical, and Supervisory Aspects of One-at-a-Time Services* (pp. 116–134). New York: Routledge.

Slive, A., & Bobele, M. (2011). *When One Hour Is All You Have: Effective Therapy for Walk-In Clients.* Phoenix, AZ: Zeig, Tucker & Theisen.

Slive, A. & Bobele, M. (2018). The three top reasons why walk-ins/single-sessions make perfect sense. In M.F. Hoyt et al. (Eds.), *Single-Session Therapy by Walk-In or Appointment: Administrative, Clinical, and Supervisory Aspects of One-at-a-Time Services* (pp. 27–39). New York: Routledge.

Slive, A., Maclaurin, B., Oakander, M., & Amundson, J. (1995). Walk-in single sessions: A new paradigm in clinical service delivery. *Journal of Systemic Therapies, 14,* 3–11.

Slive, A., McElheran, N., & Lawson, A. (2008). How brief does it get? Walk-in single session therapy. *Journal of Systemic Therapies, 27,* 5–22.

Soo-Hoo, T. (2018). Working within the client's cultural context in single-session therapy. In M.F. Hoyt et al. (Eds.), *Single-Session Therapy by Walk-In or Appointment: Administrative, Clinical, and Supervisory Aspects of One-at-a-Time Services* (pp. 186–201). New York: Routledge.

Talmon, M. (1990). *Single Session Therapy: Maximizing the Effect of the First (and Often Only) Therapeutic Encounter*. San Francisco, CA: Jossey-Bass.

Talmon, M. (1993). *Single Session Solutions: A Guide to Practical, Effective, and Affordable Therapy*. Reading, MA: Addison-Wesley.

Young, K. (2018). Change in the winds: The growth of walk-in therapy clinics in Ontario, Canada. In M.F. Hoyt et al. (Eds.), *Single-Session Therapy by Walk-In or Appointment: Administrative, Clinical, and Supervisory Aspects of One-at-a-Time Services* (pp. 59–71). New York: Routledge.

Chapter 4

Single-session therapy – past and future

An interview with Jeff Young[1]

Introduction

Single-session therapy by walk-in or appointment has, over the last few years, attracted increasing attention across the world as service providers grapple with lengthening waiting lists, pressure on public funding for services and greater community expectations for accessible, high-quality, client-led services. Single-Session Therapy (SST), which paradoxically does not preclude the client having further sessions, has become popular as a way of providing services at the point of need rather than at the point of availability. Based on international research that shows the modal number of therapeutic sessions that clients have across a wide range of presentations is one and that the majority of these clients report being satisfied with that session and decide not to seek further help (Hoyt & Talmon, 2014; Hoyt, Bobele, Slive, Young & Talmon, 2018), SST attempts to 'make the most of every encounter'. Our clients seem to be telling us something! In this interview, I (WD) interviewed Jeff Young (a leading figure in the international SST community) on his views on the past and future development of this field. This interview took place (via Skype, between London, England and Brunswick, Victoria, Australia) on 7 March 2018.[2]

> **Windy:** So, Jeff, how would you describe the impact of single-session therapy since Moshe Talmon published his book in 1990?
>
> **Jeff:** Well, Moshe's book was certainly a turning point (Talmon, 1990). Before that time, there had been a number of small independent studies and anecdotal reports that suggested a significant number of clients choose to attend only one

session and that many of these clients reported surprising results, but Moshe's book, in a very powerful way, pulled all of that research together. And I think, from that time, we went from a range of independent, radical clinical findings to the beginnings of a movement; of a paradigm shift, under the name 'single-session therapy'. Since that time, single-session therapy ideas have developed under two broad banners: single-session therapy (SST), including applying single-session thinking to different work contexts, including many tough front-line services and disaster relief; and the walk-in services that Arnie Slive and his team, in Calgary, Canada, developed also from the early 1990s.

The underlying principles have challenged conventional therapeutic service delivery and our construction of therapy and therapeutic change. The popularisation of the SST research has brought a realisation that a significant number of clients who we see will decide to 'drop out' after one session, whether we like it or not. The good news is that the research, pulled together by Moshe Talmon in 1990, revealed that whilst the most common number of sessions (the mode, not the average) clients attend is one session, the majority (68%–88%) of these clients who 'drop out' after one session actually report, when contacted, that they were satisfied with that one-off session; they are usually not 'drop outs' but satisfied customers. This and subsequent research is starting to make clinicians aware that a significant number of their clients will decide to only attend one session and that, at least for some clients, they can actually make a significant difference in that one session.

A huge challenge for clinicians, however, is that it appears we can't tell who is going to come once and who will come more often. Clinically, my colleagues and I are hopeless at predicting who will decide to do more work and who won't. Over time, we have realised this is not a problem, but it does require a major conceptual change in thinking about the first and subsequent sessions, and about therapeutic change in general. The fundamental shift we have had to make is to approach the first session 'as if' it is going to be the last, even if it isn't. This has significant ramifications for the clinician and for the service in which the clinician is working. For the clinician this means, no matter what therapeutic model you embrace, your task is to seek out what the client wants to 'walk away with at the end of the session' and then to align your focus to this goal and to work very hard to provide what the client wants. This typically involves 'checking in' from time to time to ensure you are on task and being helpful and being very generous and open about sharing your thoughts with the client. You can begin to see why the client feedback about SST is very positive (see Boyhan, 1996; Hymmen, Stalker & Cait, 2013); it is not only philosophically client-led, it is practically client-led, because the clinician is directed to addressing the client's practical goal and is dedicated to making the most of every encounter.

From the service point of view, we see clients (families) for a single session and then, if there are no risk issues, we follow up with a phone call a week or two later to collaboratively discuss whether family members want another single session, ongoing work, referral to a specialist service or to complete. I think this period post the first session, when clients are expected to try out the ideas raised in the first session, backed up by the support of the therapist and the potential for further follow-up sessions, is an ideal context for client-driven change. We tell clients that they can also contact us at any time, we always offer an 'open door'. Maybe because the door is always 'open' we find clients seldom have to knock.

Organisationally, it means providing processes to support the idea that one session may be sufficient, as determined by the client, AND at the same time to ensure there are no constraints to further work if the client wants further help. Another confronting finding from the SST literature is that clients rather than clinicians will mostly choose how many sessions they will attend.

Windy: So then what is the definition of SST, just to be clear?

Jeff: There are a number of different definitions of SST (see Hoyt, Bobele, Slive, Young & Talmon, 2018). I prefer a fundamental definition based on the research findings that led to the development of single-session work. It might be easier to quote from my chapter (Young, 2018, 44):

Single-Session Therapy [is] everything that derives attitudinally, clinically, and organizationally from accepting three findings, two backed by research and the third by our clinical experience.

Finding #1: that the most common number of service contacts that clients attend is one, followed by two, followed by three... irrespective of diagnosis, complexity, or the severity of their problem (Talmon, 1990). Finding #2: that the majority (often about 70–80% percent) of those people who attend only one session, across a range of therapies, report that the single session was adequate given their current circumstance (Talmon, 1990; Bloom, 2001; Campbell, 2012). Finding #3: possibly the hardest finding to accept, is that it seems impossible to accurately predict who will attend only one session and who will attend more, a proposition that has significant clinical and organizational ramifications.

As you can see, I define SST as a service delivery model, not as a specific model of therapy. If a clinician accepts the SST research findings it will influence how they will deliver their particular model of therapy.

In our SST workshops, we use the following guided imagery exercise to help participants to imagine what their work would look like if they were influenced by the SST research. The exercise goes something like this. No matter what model of therapy you embrace, imagine conducting a first session with a client when you and the client are expecting this session to be the first of, let's say, six sessions. Reflect on how you would typically introduce the work, build rapport, notice the questions you would ask early in the session, how you would decide what to focus on and how you would begin to finish the session, including what feedback you would share with the client, before rebooking for the second of six sessions. Then we introduce a change. We say, the morning before you conduct this session, the client informs you that they are migrating to Australia the day following your session. We then ask, re-imagine conducting this same session with the same client, but this time knowing this first session will be the last. Imagine how you would introduce the work, build rapport, notice what questions you would ask and what you would share with the client before wishing them well in Australia. Comparing the later imaginary session to the first gives clinicians unfamiliar with SST an insight into how SST thinking would influence their preferred model of therapy. Again, SST paradoxically does not restrict sessions to one, if the client decides they want further help, but, at the same time, it does entertain the real possibility that, independent of diagnosis, severity and the clinician's view, one session may be sufficient, as defined by the client.

Windy: You mentioned walk-in services – what are they and how do they relate to SST?

Jeff: Walk-ins are a different service delivery model again. No red tape, no intake criteria, no follow-up. Risk is managed as required and supported by the client being able to return for another session, again without any red tape and hence as easily as the first time. So practically it could be argued that follow-up is readily available. Once the clinician is in the room, they (and the client) approach the session knowing from the start it will be a one off, rather than 'as if' it will be the last, as in SST. Clients are welcome to re-present, but this session is also treated as another one off. Whilst walk-ins have the advantage of greater accessibility, they are harder to staff, usually requiring trainees on placement, because if multiple clients walk in at the same time, you need to have multiple clinicians available ready to respond to unpredictable demand. Woods Homes in Canada have a team of trainees ready to respond and report an average waiting time of 20 minutes before walk-in clients are seen. A disadvantage is that the possibility of planned ongoing work, which is one option post an initial session in the SST service delivery system, is not usually available.

Windy: What other key research developments have occurred since Moshe pulled the early SST research together?

Jeff: Since Moshe's book, there has been significant research. Bloom's (2001) review pulled together the research post 1990. In Australia, Alistair Campbell (2012) summarised the research post Bloom, in a special SST edition of the Australian and New Zealand *Journal of Family Therapy*, which my colleague Pam Rycroft and I co-edited. We have two textbooks based on the first two International SST conferences (Hoyt & Talmon, 2014; Hoyt et al., 2018). Really it does create a strong, not an outcome evidence-base, but a strong process evidence-base. Outcome research is difficult because SST is really a service delivery model not a specific model of therapy. Much more rigorous outcome research is required, but it needs to compare like with like – i.e. SST delivery approach of therapy 'A' compared to a normal provision of therapy 'A' – and focus on process (did fewer people drop out, were fewer sessions needed for the same outcome etc.).

What the research does say pretty clearly is that a lot of people come to therapy once, whether we like it or not. And, surprisingly, a lot of positive, useful and significant outcomes can result from that one session. And we don't know who will attend once and who will seek further help. Accepting these findings leads to the paradigm shift. It challenges the idea that complex problems always require long-term solutions; it also challenges the idea that simple problems only require brief solutions. The most significant impact of the research is that it challenges the entrenched view that the only way to achieve significant change is through deep change that can only happen through long-term work. It can happen in that way, but it can also happen in very different ways; as in one-off sessions. I think SST frees up the field to think about change and the role of therapists in promoting change in different ways.

Windy: I would say the archetype of deep change over a short period of time is Scrooge: he had three single sessions with three ghostly therapists overnight.

Jeff: Yes, ironically there are many accounts of deep personal change in response to a single (or three) significant event(s) or encounter(s) in literature, in film and in the community. But the assumption in health and welfare services, that significant therapeutic change always requires long term-work, is quite entrenched and cherished. A long-term psychotherapist in one of our early SST workshops, who was cynical that one occasion of therapy could ever lead to significant change in anyone, told me during a lunch-time discussion how he'd personally been transformed by a particular film he'd seen.

Practitioners seldom believe the SST findings until they experience them themselves usually when they seek feedback from clients who only attend one session. Irving Yalom, the internationally renowned long-term therapist, was interviewed at a family therapy conference in Australia by Paul Gibney, a local advocate of long-term therapy. The interviewer asked, 'What do you say to young therapists who are frustrated that funding cuts restrict their capacity to conduct long-term therapy?' Yalom responded, 'Well, as I have travelled the world, a lot of people come up to me and want my help and because I'm not going to be in any one city for very long, I agree to speak to them for a one-off session and it can be quite effective.' He then described the principles of single-session therapy beautifully, without knowing the SST literature.

So, for me, this is a powerful argument for single-session work, that someone who is an advocate of long-term therapy, when forced to see a client for one session, naturally found a way to adapt their longer-term approach to 'making the most of that one encounter' and was very positive and surprised about the outcome.

Windy: SST would not be suitable for all clients. Which clients would SST not be suitable for?

Jeff: I'm glad you asked this question. 'For whom is SST indicated and for whom is SST contraindicated?' was the most asked question when we started training people in SST. It was tricky to answer initially because our clinical experience was that many clients we thought would come once wanted multiple sessions when we telephoned to follow up, and some clients who had major difficulties decided that the initial session was sufficient. So, we began to develop a 'Buddhist like' non-attachment to outcome. We would try to make the most of our first session, then say to clients, we'll ring you in a week or two and ask you how you'd like to proceed; another single session, ongoing work, referral or finish. A helpful way to think about SST is that once the initial session is complete, all of the services provided by your services currently are still available to the client, with the addition of, don't laugh, 'a second single session'.

Now we have an answer to your question. The answer is, embed SST into your service system so that all options your service can provide are available to the client following the single session, and then you don't have to decide who will be satisfied with one session and who will not. As I said earlier, we have found we are hopeless at assessing who will come once and who will want more sessions. It's quite confronting initially as a professional, and then liberating. You just wait, with an open mind, and see what the client wants at the follow-up phone call.

Windy: Do you think there is anything about the context of Canada and Australia that has provided a good foundation for the development of SST or walk-in services? They're not very popular in England. I'm not sure that they are very widespread in the United States of America.

Jeff: I think it is more that you need a group of people working and promoting the work. For example, a colleague of mine, Flavio Cannistrà, has recently established the first SST Institute in Italy (see Cannistrà and Piccirilli, 2018), Martin Söderquist is currently writing a book based on his and his colleagues' work on single-session couple therapy in Malmo, Sweden, my colleagues Arnie Slive and Monte Bobele (2011) are developing walk-in services in Texas and with colleagues in Mexico. My Bouverie colleagues led by Brendan O'Hanlon have introduced Single Session Family Consultations in Alcohol and Drug Services across New Zealand (see bouverie.org.au).

At the Bouverie Centre we have 40 staff, and we have had a significant group of people working on single-session work. We have trained close to 5,000 workers from hundreds of different services over a period of 24 years. But in the early days of our training, there was great cynicism and even hostility. And I know Moshe and his team, when they started teaching SST ideas in the US, also encountered significant hostility. I don't think Woods Homes in Alberta, where walk-in services were developed, experienced any hostility, certainly not from the community, because the approach was designed in response to community consultation. The community, when asked, wanted a counselling service when they wanted it (Saturday mornings), in non-stigmatising settings (shopping centres), no red tape (no intake criteria) and easily accessed (available for walk ins).

The SST literature is quite confronting, but the early hostility was due to a misinterpretation of the approach. Practitioners thought we wanted to reduce services to clients, and, of course, that is an outrageous idea for people who are committed to good outcomes and supporting clients and people who are struggling with difficulties.

Over time we have learnt to ask participants in our workshops and people in our capacity-building projects around single-session work, 'What is your current client contact data?' I'd almost bet my house that in 90% of times or more the graph of their contact data is the same; the most common number of sessions is one, followed by two, followed by three, followed by four, with a long tail. So then, we say, 'We are not actually trying to get you to reduce resources, this is what you are doing already. We assume you want to provide a good service, not only to the few people in the long tail of the graph who come many times, but also to the people who come once or twice. You are already seeing a lot of people once or twice, let's give them the best possible service. Practitioners are more accepting of SST with this rationale.

The clinical consequences of adopting the single-session research are also very contemporary in terms of the ethics of psychotherapy. Practically, it leads to responsive, client-led, collaborative, transparent practice. Linking these practical consequences of single-session thinking to the value base of the clinicians and their organisations is very powerful. We have found that, over time, after considerable initial caution and suspicion, many practitioners and organisations embrace it.

Windy: So that's where we are at the moment. Let's switch our focus to the future. I will first ask you to predict the future, whether you like it or not, then to look at which direction you would like to see the field develop, and, finally, what developments you fear might happen, that you would prefer not to see. Does that structure make sense to you that we could follow?

Jeff: Yeah, that's fine.

Windy: So, let's start off with your predictions: what are your predictions about how you think single-session therapy will develop in the future?

Jeff: Could I preface my comments by saying one thing that has been helpful, and is probably an important development post-Talmon, is the three international single-session conferences – the inaugural one we hosted in 2012 at Phillip Island, Australia (see Hoyt & Talmon, 2014), the second one in Banff, Canada, in 2015 (see Hoyt et al., 2018) and the third one in Melbourne, Australia, in 2019 – because that does connect you with other people in the field and across nations, and you do get a sense of where things are moving or not.

So, I think SST could go in either of two ways. It could either gradually have a profound impact on the way health services are delivered clinically and organisationally across the world, which has sort of happened in our state of Victoria, and is starting to happen in other states of Australia. Or it could continue to be practised in small pockets, and many of these pockets of practice would peter out over time, with people reverting back to the usual ways of thinking about change and therapy and providing services.

I think there are a number of drivers that will make it more likely to have a broader, international impact over time. One is if the single-session therapy field itself emphasises the underlying principles, rather than aligning itself with a particular model of therapy. If the underlying principles are emphasised and the field promotes the idea that any model of therapy can be practised with a single-session attitude, that would be one driver. Seen in this way, it could be a positive disruptive influence on models of therapy that don't currently embrace a client-led collaborative transparent practice. This has the advantage that SST would align with the philosophy that modern service delivery is moving toward anyway. So that could be another driver.

Windy: Why do you say SST promotes client-led collaborative transparent practice?

Jeff: If a therapist approaches the first session 'as if' it is going to be the last, it invites that therapist, no matter what their therapeutic training is, to make overt that the session may be the last. It is a natural next step to then clarify what the client would like to achieve by the end of the session. If you and the client accept that the first session may also be the last, it provides a context for 'making the most of the time available'. I've found that making the most of the first session naturally leads the practitioner to be upfront about what the client wants to achieve and how best to achieve it. It provides a context for both therapist and client to 'cut to the chase' because they both realise that they may not have the luxury of waiting for the key issues to arise in the natural course of a conversation. SST also provides an incentive for therapists to share what they are thinking as they begin to think it, rather than accumulating a 'water tight' case over several sessions before sharing their hypothesis or advice with the client. Essentially the therapist operating under an SST approach would ask themselves, 'What would I want to share with this client if I never see them again?' Given it is not possible to be confident about a hypothesis or advice in just one session, it seems natural to co-develop the hypothesis and to share the advice in the subjunctive. For example, 'I'm beginning to get some ideas, I will share them with you and see what you think? Or tell me if I've got this totally wrong, but I'm wondering if...' Also as the clinician, you've got to take client feedback seriously and change your approach and feedback accordingly.

Windy: What other things could promote a broader uptake of SST ways of working?

Jeff: Another driver could come from greater promotion of clients' experiences of SST approaches. Clients typically rate the approach very highly as I've mentioned because of the alignment between client and worker; the collaboration and transparency that SST approaches promote.

However, maybe the most powerful driver will be an economic one. I think, over time, there is going to be growing pressure on health and welfare services to provide efficient and effective services, but at the same time services will also be confronted with fiscal pressures of the ageing population, and public funding will not be available to simply increase existing service delivery systems as need increases. Healthcare costs will have to be contained and limited. So, you'll have an empowered educated community wanting accessible, high-quality responsive services, and wanting them right now, and at the same time restricted funding will limit the proliferation of services. I think single-session thinking can inform ways to address this dilemma and provide part of a way forward. We know from experience that if services provide immediate, one-off sessions while also providing a pathway for longer, more intensive work, waiting lists tend to reduce. And we know that clients really love this type of service delivery because clinicians are not only ideologically putting clients in the driver's seat; if they approach the first session 'as if' it is the last, they practically have to put clients in the driver's seat.

So that's how I hope it goes, because I think then the SST paradigm shift could potentially have an impact not only on clinicians, but on the community. It could be used to change the community's view of counselling.

Windy: So it is almost as if you are saying that, in parallel with clinicians developing a single-session mindset, the community learns to adopt a single-session mindset as well.

Jeff: Yes. It's like with your work, where you've publicly done single-session interventions for both professionals and community members. That is an example of promoting the idea that a lot of people can be helped in one session, if it's done well. And I like your work, although we come from different models of practice – me a family therapist, you a cognitive behavioural therapist – which in itself is an example of how single-session therapy can unite practitioners across different models of practice. Promoting SST approaches can potentially create opportunities for the community to learn that therapy is not that scary, and you can actually have brief encounters that can be helpful. You can get back on track and you can even do it publicly because it's non-blaming and it's non-judgemental. It's a very positive approach to people and their problems. Therapy presented in this way may lead people in the community to think, 'If I don't have to commit to longer-term work, I might actually try it, and then I might suggest my friend try it too, because he or she is in a bit of trouble at the moment.'

And, maybe in parallel to that, the managers, funders and directors of services may start to think, 'Actually, single-session inspired services can be an efficient way to help more people and to help services be more accessible, and there's pressure on us to do that.'

Windy: So, in a way, it sounds like your predictions dovetail, at the moment, with what you'd like to see.

Jeff: Well, I guess I'm saying it could go either way. That would be the way that I would like it to go, but it could go both ways.

Windy: What is the other way?

Jeff: The field could also fall into the trap of attaching SST to a particular model; creating competition about which model of single-session therapy works best. SST approaches could continue to be practised in small pockets that are isolated and not connected with each other. Over time, we have seen organisations that have fully implemented an SST approach, the clinicians and clients love it, then, five years later, it has vanished without a trace.

So, I think we need to start with building on the international networks that have resulted from the first two conferences. The third one was in October 2019 in Melbourne, Australia. The theme was 'SST (Single Session Thinking); going global one step at a time'. There we were able to continue to build international connections, promote collaborative research and strong implementation strategies. The fact that SST is implementable, because you are not teaching an alternative therapeutic model, just how the clinician can deliver their current therapeutic model in an SST way, is another SST strength. I have already mentioned that the Bouverie Centre has led a number of successful SST implementation projects across state-wide organisations and services. For example, we trained all 330 counsellors and provided implementation support to all of the community health counselling services across Victoria (see Young, Weir & Rycroft, 2012) and at follow-up 49% of those services had adopted a single-session approach as a service delivery model, and 84% of clinicians reported using it in their work. When you look at the implementation research – that is an unusually high implementation rate.

Windy: So, it is almost like you are saying that the danger is, in some ways, that it becomes a fad; it galvanises people, you go back five years later, that sort of enthusiasm and excitement is no longer there.

Jeff: Yes.

Windy: So, there is a real danger. I guess that one of the ways of keeping people galvanised and interested is through these conferences, both international and local.

Jeff: Yes, and from the first conference we established a virtual community of practice (https://www.bouverie.org.au/support-for-services/communities-of-practice) and we probably haven't done that as well as we could, but I think now that should be developed further to promote international conversations. It is interesting that we have seen, at a local level in Victoria, the potential of a sustained, wide-spread implementation, but, from the second International Symposium on SST and Walk-in Therapy in Banff, in September of 2015, I realised, like you were saying earlier, that in most areas around the world SST is very small and is not having a big influence. It is still an emerging idea and one that we tried to further at the third conference.

Windy: Have you managed to be so successful in Victoria because you and other people have got the ear of politicians who are flexible and open to new ideas? Or do you think that you have managed to actually progress this stuff without that political networking?

Jeff: We have reasonably good connections, but we haven't got connections at the highest level of government. Probably Canada is starting to do that with the walk-ins more successfully than us. We have developed it with smaller projects leading to bigger projects, with the support of people at a middle management level in government who are responsible for workforce and capacity-building in state-wide services. But I think there is potential for engaging the highest level of government. I guess, in the early days, there was some reluctance from us to engage at a high political level, in case the SST research was used as an excuse to reduce services. So, we have to really explain that it is not about curing everything in a one-off session; it is not about replacing longer-term work; it is about aligning clinicians and their service delivery with the natural help-seeking behaviour of clients and with what they want.

Windy: So, you are reflecting what is happening. You are not trying to force what is happening into a particular mould. You are responding to what is happening naturally, and really saying, 'Let's help people get the most out of what they come for.'

Jeff: Yes, and then, if you do that, then services become more efficient, but not at the expense of what clients want. Clients are getting what they want, when they need it, and in the way that they want it, so then they become more engaged and the work becomes more efficient and more effective. So, this is the way I think single-session thinking can help services address funding challenges, not by simply cutting services.

What really helped our implementation of SST in the community health counselling services across Victoria was the original client contact data. For the three years prior to our single-session training, of a total of 104,000 clients, 42% had come once, 18% had come twice, and 10% came three times. So, we are able to use their own data to say, 'Well, this is what's already happening. We know you, the clinicians, want to provide the best possible service to the 42% of those 104,000 clients who currently only attend one session.' That was very compelling. But we were also saying, 'We also want to give the best possible outcome for the people who come six times, as well as those who come 10, 20, 30 times.' Community health counsellors are very political and that argument, when they realised it also led to putting clients in charge of the work, was a sensible rationale for them that aligned with their values.

Windy: Do you have any other fears about how single-session therapy may develop?

Jeff: I guess one of my greatest fears is that people take the words in the title verbatim and think that the goal of a single-session service or the goal of a single-session clinician is to cure in one session. That is unrealistic and would put undue pressure on clients, and on clinicians. It is, in my view, a misinterpretation of the research underlying SST.

Windy: One of the things that Albert Ellis said towards the end of his life about the name of 'Rational Emotive Behaviour Therapy' was, 'I think I made a mistake calling it rational, because people hear "rational" and then they turn off.' Nobody stepped up to the plate and said, 'Well, look, let's get rid of the word "rational". It's turning people off.' It is almost as if I get a sense, when I speak to you and to other people in the field, that there is a saying, 'We're stuck with this term now, which, if we were to name it where we are now, we wouldn't have called it single-session therapy; we would've called it one-at-a-time therapy,' which is another alternative name. Am I picking that up from you?

Jeff: I've explored this with colleagues here and around the world many times (see Young, 2018), and I've come to the conclusion it is both a huge advantage for the field and a great curse. The term is so in your face that, in a way, it is a great publicity tool. If we called it one-at-a-time therapy, we wouldn't be where we are now. Because it was called single-session therapy, and especially if I reflect back to the early days, people would come to our workshops almost to give us a hard time about the title. But we would see this amazing transformative shift in the workshops where angry cynical participants would go away once they really understood the concept, that it was client-led and empowering to clients, and become real advocates of the approach. But, at the same time, it's a misnomer and doesn't really reflect the nuance of the underlying paradigm.

I don't know about you, Windy, but to me and my colleagues here at Bouverie, it has been a real challenge to articulate and define SST precisely. On one level, it is so simple, and yet it is very hard to define.

Windy: If I was going to say what one of my hopes is, the features that we have been discussing become, in a sense, not just attached to this strange thing called single-session therapy, but it becomes the foundation for good clinical work, whether it be with families, couples, CBT, narrative therapy, or whatever. In a sense, because the naturally occurring pattern, as you pointed out, is one followed by two, etc., then people are being trained to do the very work that they actually do.

Jeff: Yes. I would have a very similar hope to that. In the past, therapists would commonly see someone, and if the client didn't come back after one session the therapist would assume either the client or they had failed. And because there was no overt discussion about whether the client needed to come back or not, or whether that one session may be enough, if things improved after the first session, the client just wouldn't show up again. They wouldn't contact to say, 'Thanks, the session helped, I may see you in the future but I'm ok for now.' Clinicians incorrectly called those people 'dropouts' and much worse. Baekeland and Lundwall (1975) reviewed 330 articles on how therapists described people who had dropped out after one session, and they tended to use surprisingly pejorative language. A negative consequence of this is that clients who 'drop out' because the first session was helpful may feel embarrassed about re-contacting the service if they need help in the future.

I think it is a fascinating question, 'what has been the impact on the field and on clinicians that one of the most common outcomes (one-off sessions) in counselling has been viewed as a failure?' I think clinicians, depending on their locus of control, would either have blamed clients for not being good clients or blamed themselves for not being good therapists, when, in actual fact, it was both very common and, in most cases, a good outcome.

In different contexts it translates differently, but the way we translate single-session thinking into our counselling context is that we inform clients from the start that we will make the most of the first session, people have the session, and we don't make the decision on whether the client comes back or not in the session. If there are no risk issues, we encourage a phone call down the track to see whether they want to come back. The period between the first session and the phone call provides a rich context for change. We have suggested some ideas for change in the session, now it is over to you, but help is only a phone call away. The follow-up phone call also gives us information and feedback about how useful the session was, and whether people want further help or not. It institutionalises what, as you say, actually happens; that people might often feel that one is enough and, rather than seeing them as dropouts, or the session as a failure, you say, 'That's fantastic, feel free to come back if you want to anytime.' So it opens up opportunities for both, and this is the nuanced approach that one session may be enough, but, if it's not, you can come back, even in a year's time, and you don't have to feel embarrassed because you didn't drop out; we actually agreed and it was all upfront that one session was enough at the time. So, it potentially creates a really transparent, healthy, normal service delivery system that can help demystify counselling. This is its potential. I am sounding a bit grandiose now but, even at a basic level, single-session thinking can help align service delivery with clients' natural help-seeking behaviour.

Notes

1 Jeff Young (PhD) is the Director of The Bouverie Centre: Victoria's Family Institute, La Trobe University. His most recent publication on SST is: Young, J. (2018). Single-Session Therapy: The gift that keeps on giving. In M.F. Hoyt, M. Bobele, A. Slive, J. Young & M. Talmon

(Eds.), *Single-Session Therapy by Walk-In or Appointment: Clinical, Supervisory, and Administrative Aspects*. New York: Routledge.

2 I made some modifications to the transcript on 24/03/20.

References

Baekeland, F., & Lundwall, L. (1975). Dropping out of treatment: A critical review. *Psychological Bulletin, 82*(5), 738–783.

Bloom, B.L. (2001). Focused single session psychotherapy: A review of the clinical and research literature. *Brief Treatment and Crisis Intervention, 1*(1), 75–86.

Boyhan, P. (1996). Clients' perceptions of single session consultations as an option to waiting for family therapy. *Australian and New Zealand Journal of Family Therapy, 17*(2), 85–96.

Campbell, A. (2012). Single-session approaches to therapy: Time to review. *Australian and New Zealand Journal of Family Therapy, 33*(1), 15–26.

Cannistrà, F., & Piccirilli, F. (Eds.) (2018). *Manuale italiano di terapia a seduta singola*. Firenze: Giunti.

Hoyt, M.F., & Talmon, M.F. (2014). What the literature says: An annotated bibliography. In M.F. Hoyt & M. Talmon (Eds.), *Capturing the Moment: Single Session Therapy and Walk-In Services* (pp. 487–516). Bethel, CT: Crown House Publishing.

Hoyt, M.F., Bobele, M., Slive, A., Young, J., & Talmon, M. (Eds.) (2018). *Single-Session Therapy by Walk-In or Appointment: Clinical, Supervisory, and Administrative Aspects*. New York: Routledge.

Hymmen, P., Stalker, C.A., & Cait, C. (2013). The case for single-session therapy: Does the empirical evidence support the increased prevalence of this service delivery model and walk-in services? *Journal of Mental Health, 22*(1), 60–71.

Slive, A., & Bobele, M. (Eds.) (2011). *When One Hour Is All You Have: Effective Therapy for Walk-In Clients*. Phoenix, AZ: Zeig, Tucker & Theisen.

Talmon, M. (1990). *Single Session Therapy: Maximizing the Effect of the First (and Often Only) Therapeutic Encounter*. San Francisco, CA: Jossey-Bass.

Young, J. (2018). Single Session Therapy: The gift that keeps on giving. In M.F. Hoyt, M. Bobele, A. Slive, J. Young, & M. Talmon (Eds.), *Single-Session Therapy by Walk-In or Appointment: Clinical, Supervisory, and Administrative Aspects* (pp. 40–58). New York: Routledge.

Young, J., Weir, S., & Rycroft, P. (2012). Implementing single session therapy. *Australian and New Zealand Journal of Family Therapy, 33*(1), 84–97.

Chapter 5

The future of single-session therapy

A synthesis

Overview

In Chapters 2–4, I interviewed three key figures in the SST field: Moshe Talmon from Israel, Michael Hoyt from the USA, and Jeff Young from Australia.[1] I asked them for their predictions about the future of SST and about their hopes and fears for that future. In this closing chapter, I synthesise Talmon's, Hoyt's and Young's responses and put forward a collective view of the future of single-session therapy.

Predictions about the future of SST

Moshe Talmon chose not to answer the question about predictions, citing the famous quotation, 'predictions are for fools'.[2] By contrast, both Michael Hoyt and Jeff Young – although neither of them are fools – responded to this question. Hoyt predicted that more therapists would practise SST going forward and particularly within a walk-in context. He also thought that its practice would increase over the Internet, but that this would raise issues of jurisdiction and licensure. Finally, he predicted that, in addition to an increase in the practice of SST, there would also be an increase in publications and training.

Young suggested that the future of SST could go in one of two directions. On a positive note, with the support of international collaborations in research, training and implementation, he thought it could increasingly have a significant impact on the way health services are delivered clinically and organisationally across the world. He thought there would be two broad drivers for this. First, practitioners would see that they could practise SST within their own orientation and that it was not inextricably linked to any specific therapeutic approach. The more SST is seen as a mindset rather than an approach, the more this is likely to happen. Consistently high levels of SST client satisfaction (Hymmen, Stalker & Cait, 2013) would further promote its acceptance. Second, there would be an economic driver for this development. With ageing populations and decreasing healthcare budgets, if money was invested in providing a quick, accessible, client-led response to therapeutic need, along with the fact that many of these contacts would be single sessions and that most clients would be satisfied with such contact, then such investment would be seen as being well spent which, especially if these timely responses reduced costs in other areas of the health budget, would lead to further investment. As long as this did not mean that further help, if needed, was withheld, then this would herald a promising future for SST and walk-in services.

On the other hand, Young said that SST could have a less promising future where it would be seen just as a specific approach and not as a general mindset. Consequently, it could become a fading fad and be practised in smaller and smaller circles as those initially enthusiastic about SST gradually moved away from it. People would then revert back to older and more traditional ways of thinking about therapy and of service provision.

Hopes for the future of SST

Talmon hoped that single-session therapy would be integrated with all services, with various approaches to therapy (as did Hoyt and Young) and in diverse settings. He also hoped that, while still being evidence-based, SST would be individually tailored to each client rather than be protocol driven. Finally, he hoped that SST would be utilised in 'advanced systems' (such as artificial intelligence and social media) to encourage people to connect together directly and to get help quickly, but without losing its human presence.

Hoyt's hopes centred on the universal availability of SST, especially for those who couldn't afford regular therapy. He further hoped that more attention would be paid in the provision of SST to cultural nuances and that SST would capitalise on recent developments in strengths-based therapy to place more emphasis on bringing forward people's abilities.

Young hoped that his positive predictions as outlined above would be realised, thus assisting the healthcare industry to respond to the growing community expectation of efficient, collaborative, consumer-led, transparent service delivery.

Fears about the future of SST

All of my interviewees voiced their fears that data on the effectiveness of SST and walk-in therapy would be used by government agencies and insurance companies to restrict people to one session irrespective of their need for further services. Related to this, Talmon expressed his concern that this 'one size fits all' extrapolation from the quantitative and qualitative research literature on SST would lead 'to a narrowing or flattening of human struggle and human suffering'.

Echoing Young's less promising future (outlined above), Hoyt feared that SST might become just a particular approach rather than a more general mindset, although he was open to the possibility that research might show that specific SST approaches might be specifically helpful for specific problems. He also expressed concern that some people would have the unrealistic expectation that all problems could be resolved in one visit.

Young also said that one of his greatest fears was that the SST paradigm would be misinterpreted in that people would take the term 'single-session therapy' literally and think that the goal of a single-session service or the goal of a single-session clinician was to cure in one session. If this happened, it would place undue pressure on both clients and therapists and would strip SST of its potency and of its place as an integral part of a broader service provision.

Epilogue

This brings us to the end of the book. I hope you have found it of interest and it has stimulated your thinking about single-session therapy and how it might develop. Perhaps Moshe Talmon was correct not to make predictions about the future of SST. For who was to know in late 2018 when I conducted the interviews that the world only two years later would be in the grip of the Coronavirus and that face-to-face therapy sessions would be suspended worldwide to prevent infection? And yet such is the flexibility of the SST mindset and way of delivering services that it might prove an excellent way of providing therapeutic services to communities fearful about the future of their world and perhaps of *the* world. Certainly, its practitioners have shown such flexibility in dealing with other world crises and disasters (see Hoyt & Talmon, 2014; Hoyt, Bobele, Slive, Young & Talmon, 2018). When the dust settles and the world eventually returns to a semblance of 'normality', we will see if the hopes of Talmon, Hoyt and Young have been realised.

Notes

1 I would again like to thank Michael Hoyt, Moshe Talmon and Jeff Young for the generous gift of their time in agreeing to be interviewed and for reviewing the transcripts of the interviews.
2 The actual quotation is "Only a fool would make predictions, especially about the future" and is attributed to movie mogul Samuel Goldwyn. Hoyt also expressed caution about how accurately one can foretell events, given all the impinging contingencies, and quoted the American writer Mark Twain who said, "I don't like to make predictions, especially about the future."

References

Hoyt, M.F., & Talmon, M.F. (Eds.) (2014). *Capturing the Moment: Single Session Therapy and Walk-In Services*. Bethel, CT: Crown House Publishing.

Hoyt, M.F., Bobele, M., Slive, A., Young, J., & Talmon, M. (Eds.) (2018). *Single-Session Therapy by Walk-In or Appointment: Clinical, Supervisory, and Administrative Aspects*. New York: Routledge.

Hymmen, P., Stalker, C.A., & Cait, C. (2013). The case for single-session therapy: Does the empirical evidence support the increased prevalence of this service delivery model and walk-in services? *Journal of Mental Health*, 22(1), 60–71.

Index

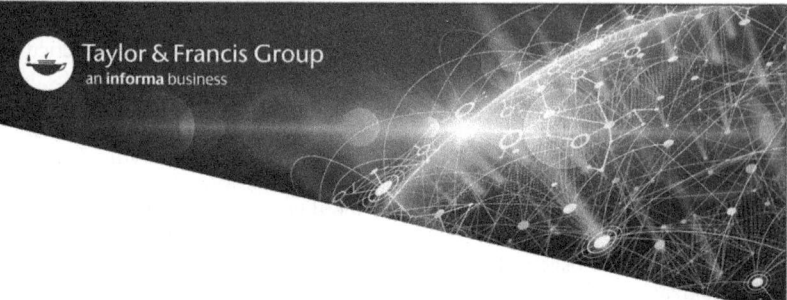
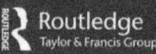
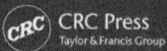